Essential Oils for Healing

A Beginners Guide to Uses and Blends

© **Copyright 2024 - All rights reserved.**

The content contained within this book may not be reproduced, duplicated or transmitted without direct written permission from the author or the publisher.

Under no circumstances will any blame or legal responsibility be held against the publisher, or author, for any damages, reparation, or monetary loss due to the information contained within this book, either directly or indirectly.

Legal Notice:

This book is copyright protected. It is only for personal use. You cannot amend, distribute, sell, use, quote or paraphrase any part, or the content within this book, without the consent of the author or publisher.

Disclaimer Notice:

Please note the information contained within this document is for educational and entertainment purposes only. All effort has been executed to present accurate, up to date, reliable, complete information. No warranties of any kind are declared or implied. Readers acknowledge that the author is not engaged in the rendering of legal, financial, medical or professional advice. The content within this book has been derived from various sources. Please consult a licensed professional before attempting any techniques outlined in this book.

By reading this document, the reader agrees that under no circumstances is the author responsible for any losses, direct or indirect, that are incurred as a result of the use of the information contained within this document, including, but not limited to, errors, omissions, or inaccuracies.

Table of Contents

INTRODUCTION 1

CHAPTER 1: ESSENTIAL OIL BASICS 3
   WHAT ARE ESSENTIAL OILS AND HOW ARE THEY MADE? 3
      History and Origins 4
      The Science Behind Essential Oils and Their Efficacy 5
      Essential Oils vs Carrier Oils: What's the Difference? 5
      Defining Top, Middle, and Base Notes 7
   SCIENTIFIC NAMES VS COMMON NAMES 8
   HOW TO RECOGNIZE QUALITY ESSENTIAL OILS 12

CHAPTER 2: SAFETY CONSIDERATIONS AND PRECAUTIONS TO KNOW BEFORE YOU CREATE YOUR FIRST BLEND 15
   HOW SAFE ARE ESSENTIAL OILS FOR DIFFERENT DEMOGRAPHICS? 15
      Symptoms of Toxicity to Be Aware Of 17
      Side Effects to Be Familiar With 18
      How to Tell if You're Allergic to Essential Oils 18
      How to Treat an Essential Oil Allergy Reaction 18
   TOP SAFETY PRECAUTIONS TO CONSIDER 19

CHAPTER 3: GETTING STARTED: EQUIPMENT, APPLICATIONS, BLENDING, AND STORAGE 23
   TOP ESSENTIAL OILS FOR YOUR STARTER KIT 23
   EQUIPMENT NEEDED TO BLEND YOUR OILS 26
   TOP APPLICATIONS OF COMMON ESSENTIAL OILS 28
   BLENDING AND DILUTION GUIDELINES 30
      Handy Blending Chart 31
      Rules for Blending Essential Oils 32
      Blending Classifications 32
      Safe Dilution Guidelines 34
   MEASUREMENT CONVERSION TABLE 35
   STORAGE TIPS TO KEEP IN MIND 36
   SHELF LIFE CONSIDERATIONS 37
      Do Essential Oils Expire? 38
      Simple Ways to Extend the Shelf Life of Essential Oils 38
      Shelf Life of Common Essential Oils 39
      What to Do With "Expired" Essential Oils 41

CHAPTER 4: ADVANCED BLENDING TECHNIQUES 43

- Advanced Blending Techniques 43
  - Blending by Effect 43
  - Blending by Fragrance 46
  - Blending by Note 48
  - Basic Blending Tips to Consider 49
- Unconventional Essential Oils and Blends 50
- Synergy Blends 51
  - What Are Synergy Oils? 51
  - How Do Synergy Oils Work? 52
  - Tips to Effectively Use Synergy Oils 55

CHAPTER 5: THERAPEUTIC BENEFITS OF ESSENTIAL OILS 57

- Are Essential Oils a Suitable Alternative to Medicine? 57
- Most Common Ailments That Can Be Treated With Essential Oils 59
- Recipe Blends and the Best Ways to Apply Them for the Most Common Ailments 60
  - Blend # 1: Headache Blend 60
  - Blend # 2: On-The-Go Headache Blend 61
  - Blend #3: Insect Shield 62
  - Blend #4: Sunburn Relief 62
  - Blend #5: Winter Immunity Booster 63
  - Blend #6: Peaceful Sleep Blend 64
  - Blend #7: Body Pain Relief 65
  - Blend #8: Essential Oil Chest Rub 66
  - Blend #9: Diffuser Cough Blend 67
- Tips to Integrate Essential Oil Blends Into Your Wellness Routine 67

CHAPTER 6: USING ESSENTIAL OIL BLENDS AROUND THE HOME AND OFFICE .. 75

- The Benefits of Using Essential Oils Around the Home 75
- Top Tips and Recipes to Use Essential Oils Around Every Part of Your Home 77
  - Tip #1: Use Essential Oils to Clean Counters and Surfaces 77
  - Tip #2: Add Cotton Balls to Your Cupboards 78
  - Tip #3: Add to the Tumble-Dryer to Fragrance Your Clothes and Linens 79
  - Tip #4: Refresh Your Carpets 79
  - Tip #5: Eliminate Pet Odors 80
  - Tip #6: Create Your Own Air Freshener 81
  - Tip #7: Add a Blend to Your Vacuum Cleaner 81
  - Tip #9: Eliminate Tobacco Odors 83
  - Tip #10: Create a Window Cleaning Solution 83
  - Tip #11: Restore Wooden Furniture 84
  - Tip #12: Revive the Grout in Your Floor and Wall Tiles 85
  - Tip #13: Freshen Your Mattress 86
  - Tip #14: Neutralize Bathroom Odors 86

Tip #15: Freshen Your Shoes 87
Tip #16: Remove Mold and Mildew 88
USING ESSENTIAL OILS TO REPEL BUGS AROUND YOUR HOME 89
How Do Essential Oils Deter Pests? 89
USING ESSENTIAL OILS AROUND THE OFFICE OR WORKSPACE 95
Top Reasons to Use Essential Oils in Your Workspace (And the Blends to Help You Do It) 95

CHAPTER 7: ESSENTIAL OIL MISTAKES TO AVOID AND TROUBLESHOOTING BLENDING MISHAPS 101

ESSENTIAL OIL MISTAKES TO AVOID 101
Mistake #1: Not Taking the Time to Learn About Essential and Carrier Oils 102
Mistake #2: Buying Poor-Quality Oils 102
Mistake #3: Not Using a Carrier Oil 103
Mistake #4: Running Your Diffuser All Day and Night 103
Mistake #5: Leaving the Lids Off the Essential Oils 104
Mistake #6: Using Your Pointer Finger to Dab On Your Blend 104
Mistake #7: Ingesting Essential or Carrier Oils 105
Mistake #8: Forgetting That Some Oils Can Stain 105
Mistake #9: Applying Oils That Are Photosensitive and Then Going Outside 105
Mistake #10: Using Oils and Blends Around Your Pets 106
TROUBLESHOOTING ESSENTIAL OIL BLENDING OR APPLICATION ISSUES 106
Troubleshooting Tip #1: My Blend Is Burning My Skin 107
Troubleshooting Tip #2: My Blend Is Giving Me a Rash 108
Troubleshooting Tip #3: I Accidentally Got Oil in My Eye 109
Troubleshooting Tip #4: My Essential/Carrier Oil Has Stained My Clothes 110
Troubleshooting Tip #5: My Blends Don't Seem to Be Working 111

CHAPTER 8: HANDY INDEX TABLE 115

CONCLUSION 127

Understanding the Basics 127
Heed the Precautions 128
Getting Started 128
Choose the Right Technique 128
Therapeutic Benefits 129
So Many Home Uses 129
Beginners Mistakes 129
Handy Index Table 129
And Lastly 130

ABOUT THE AUTHOR 131

REFERENCES 133

Introduction

It doesn't get much greener than essential oils: when used correctly, they are among Mother Nature's most potent remedies. –Amy Leigh Mercree

Essential oils have been around for a remarkably long time. Despite the advancements in modern medicine, essential oils are still popular for their holistic and natural approach to treating common ailments and promoting overall well-being. And since there are so many different oils to use for everything from a mild headache to treating stomach cramps, knowing where to start can be quite challenging. If you're new to the exciting world of essential oils and aromatherapy, then you know exactly what I'm talking about.

The challenge starts with learning the names and the general composition of these oils—not to mention their application methods. Then, there's mastering the whole blending process and knowing what safety precautions to be aware of. Fortunately, I've been in your shoes, and the good news is that mastering the art of creating different essential oil blends is easier than you may think!

My easy-to-understand guide here is going to cut through the complexity and offer you direction into the basics of essential oils, along with blending techniques, and application requirements. As a beginner, these tips and guidelines are going to help you create the perfect blend combinations, helping you deal with a host of ailments, and providing you with the holistic approach to healing you've been looking for.

Furthermore, I'm eager to share my own personal journey of how I used essential oils to enhance the quality of my life. Indeed, I've used oils to deal with everything from chronic headaches to improving my mood after a challenging period of grief. From my own experiences, I can honestly say that adding the right essential oil blends to your medicine cabinet is one of the best things you can do to improve your general well-being.

Again, if you're new to the essential oils scene, this guide is exactly what you need. From a brief overview of essential oil basics to the equipment you'll need to create the perfect blends, it's all right here for you. There'll also be a handy oil and ailment chart that you can use to identify the oils you need for various ailments. And in addition to all that, I will also be sharing the recipes and blending tips needed to create your first collection of essential oil blends! I hope you're as excited to embark on this wonderful journey as I am to share it with you.

So, with that said, let's jump right into Chapter 1, where I'll share some essential oil basics, such as the sciences that make them work and the differences between the top, middle, and base note oils. Last but not least, I'll also share the importance of using quality oils—and how to recognize quality oils in the first place!

Chapter 1:

Essential Oil Basics

Aromatherapy is extremely useful. If you want to go to sleep at night, and you have an aroma that calms your mind, it will help you sleep. –Deepak Chopra

Getting started on your journey to creating the perfect essential oil blends isn't quite as simple as buying the cheapest oils and mixing up a batch. Rather, it involves having an understanding of what oils actually are, how they work, and even how to identify a quality oil from a cheaper, less effective variation. Furthermore, where did using essential oils originate? And what are the common names for all those long scientific terms you may have seen on some recipes? Well, let's find out.

What Are Essential Oils and How Are They Made?

If you want to know what essential oils are in one simple sentence, it would be this: Essential oils are liquefied versions of different plants. Easy enough to wrap your mind around, right? However, it's a little more complex than that. Typically, essential oils are made using different parts of a plant to create an oil that can be used on its own or as part of a blend (a mixture of two or more oils) for its aromatic and healing properties.

Here are some simple steps that break down how oils are made:

- Select the right plant material.
- Harvest the plants.

- Prepare the plant material.

- Extract the oil by using one of the following extraction methods: steaming, water distillation, CO_2 extraction, solvent extraction, maceration, enfleurage, or cold press extraction.

- Separate the essential oil from the plant material.

- Filter and purify the mixture.

- Test and ensure that quality control is done.

- Bottle and package the oil.

Fortunately, you don't have to go through this whole process just to find the best essential oils to use in your blends or applications. Indeed, thanks to a surge of interest in natural remedies and aromatherapy, ready-made essential oils are more readily available to everyday folks. And with the recipes and tips I'll be sharing throughout this guide, you'll be able to easily create the blends needed on your journey, as well as understand the power of aromatherapy and the various methods of oil application.

History and Origins

As I mentioned in the Introduction, essential oils have been around for what seems like forever. Once referred to as "aromatic oils," essential oils have been used in many forms by many cultures. Historical evidence has tracked their first use to Lascaux in the French region of Dordogne, where cave drawings actually show how ancient civilizations would use plants for healing purposes.

More modern references date to ancient Egypt, where recorded history shows this civilization using aromatic oils for a wide range of applications. The most famous of their blends was "*Kyphi*," an aromatic oil made up of 16 oil and herb ingredients that they often used as medicine, perfume, and incense. Other countries such as China, Greece, and India also have traceable recordings of their ancestors using essential oils for medicinal purposes. In fact, many of these are still being used today.

The Science Behind Essential Oils and Their Efficacy

In short, essential oils work by interacting with your body in a ton of different ways. The most effective of these happens when you inhale essential oil *aromas*. Inhalation enables the oils to stimulate different areas of your limbic system. By helping to control physiological functions such as blood pressure, breathing, and heart rate, the correct application of an essential oil can have a remarkably positive effect on your overall health.

Some common health claims associated with applying essential oils include the following:

- reducing stress
- improving skin conditions
- aiding in digestion
- treating headaches
- boosting immunity
- improving mood

And if these aren't fascinating enough on their own, we'll also be taking a more in-depth look at the various ways essential oils can benefit your health in Chapter 5.

Essential Oils vs Carrier Oils: What's the Difference?

If you've already started reading through recipes and tips on how to create essential oil blends, then you have more than likely seen references to *carrier* oils. But what are these, exactly? And how do they differ from essential oils?

In the wonderful world of essential oil blends and natural remedies, both carrier oils and essential oils play some key roles. As you get ready to make your first blend, though, be sure not to mix the two up. To clarify the distinction, here's what you need to know:

- **Essential oils:** As I've already mentioned, essential oils are powerful concentrated extracts from different parts of plants such as flowers, leaves, roots, and stems. They are used in small quantities and often need to be diluted.

- **Carrier oils:** Commonly referred to as "base oils," carrier oils are extracted from the fatty portions of flowers and plants such as seeds, kernels, and nuts. Typically, carrier oils aren't concentrated and have very light aromas. These oils are therefore used to dilute essential oils, which in turn makes them safe for direct skin application. Since carrier oils contain fatty acids and an assortment of vitamins and minerals, they can protect and even nourish your skin. Commonly used carrier oils include the following:
    - argan oil
    - avocado oil
    - castor oil
    - almond oil
    - grapeseed oil
    - jojoba oil
    - rosehip oil
    - olive oil
    - hemp seed oil

Defining Top, Middle, and Base Notes

Now, you may have also seen references to top, middle, and base notes. So, what exactly are these references, and how do they influence the blends you're going to be making?

Well, typically, classifying essential oils into these three categories helps the user understand how volatile each oil is. Knowing how different essential oils fit into these categories will help you choose the right ones to help you create the perfect blend for whatever application you have in mind. Better yet, it will also reduce the likelihood of mixing the wrong oils and creating useless blends. Let's explore this a bit further:

- **Top:** Often referred to as "head notes," top notes have minute, light molecules that evaporate very quickly. These are the components you'll likely notice first when you open a bottle of essential oil. Furthermore, these generally comprise 10–30% of the blends you create. With light aromas, they are often the most uplifting and are also generally less expensive than middle or base oils. Here are a few common examples of the top notes:

    - basil
    - coriander
    - eucalyptus
    - lavender
    - lemon
    - tea tree

- **Middle:** Also called "heart notes," the middle notes are the scents that emerge immediately after the top notes have evaporated. These oils are usually extracted from herbs and spices. And since middle notes give a blend its main body, it's always recommended to start your blending process with it. The most common of these include the following:

- cinnamon
- citronella
- clove
- geranium
- jasmine
- ylang-ylang

- **Base notes:** As heavier oils, base notes evaporate slower than other, lighter oils. They also create the full body of the overall fragrance. These oils are extracted from the bark, roots, and other parts of trees. As a result, this tree component provides a richer, more robust fragrance. Below are a few common options here:
  - cassia
  - cedarwood
  - frankincense
  - ginger
  - myrrh
  - patchouli

Scientific Names vs Common Names

One of the most frustrating aspects of learning about essential oils is that some articles and recipes use longer, more complex scientific names, while others opt for the more common, everyday ones. Also, many bottle labels feature scientific names too! In short, if you're using the recipes that opt for the scientific names, then you're likely constantly Googling what type of oil you're supposed to be using.

It's with this very aspect in mind that I've decided to create the list below. Here, you have 45 of the most common essential oils and their scientific (botanical) names. If I do say so myself, this should make the process of finding the right oil much easier!

	Common Name	**Scientific (Botanical Name)**	**Category**
1.	Anise	Pimpinella anisum	Top
2.	Argan	Argania Spinosa	Base
3.	Arnica	Arnica montana	Base
4.	Avocado	Persea gratissima	Base
5.	Basil	Ocimum basilicum	Top
6.	Bergamont	Citrus bergamia	Top
7.	Cardamom	Elettaria cardamomum	Middle
8.	Cedarwood	Cedrus atlantica	Middle
9.	Chamomile, mixta	Chamaemelum mixtum	Middle
10.	Cinnamon bark	Cinnamomum verum	Middle
11.	Citronella	Cymbopogon nardus	Middle

12.	Coconut	Cocus nucifera	Base
13.	Clove	Syzygium aromaticum	Middle
14.	Dill	Anethum graveolens	Middle
15.	Eucalyptus	Eucalyptus globulus	Top/middle
16.	Fennel	Foeniculum vulgare	Top/middle
17.	Frankincense (Olibanum)	Boswellia carterii	Base
18.	Geranium	Pelargonium graveolens	Middle
19.	Ginger	Zingiber officinale	Middle/base
20.	Grapefruit	Citrus x paradisi	Top
21.	Jasmine	Jasminum officinale	Middle
22.	Jojoba	Simmomdsia	Base
23.	Juniper	Juniperus osteosperma and/or J. scoluporum	Middle
24.	Lavender	Lavandula angustifolia, CT Linalol	Top/middle
25.	Lemon	Citrus limon	Top
26.	Mandarin	Citrus reticulata	Top

27.	Marjoram	Origanum majorana	Middle/top
28.	Melaleuca (tea tree)	Melaleuca alternifolia	Middle
29.	Melissa (lemon balm)	Melissa officinalis	Middle/top
30.	Myrrh	Commiphora myrrha	Middle/base
31.	Nutmeg	Myristica fragrans	Top/middle
32.	Oregano	Origanum vulgare, CT Carvacrol	Middle
33.	Patchouly	Pogostemon cablin	Base
34.	Peppermint	Mentha piperita	Top
35.	Rosehip	Rosa canina	Middle
36.	Rosewood	Aniba rosaeodora	Middle
37.	Sage	Salvia officinalis	Base
38.	Sandalwood	Santalum album	Base
39.	Tarragon	Artemisia dracunculus	Middle
40.	Turmeric	Curcuma longa	Base
41.	Valerian	Valeriana officinalis	Top
42.	Vanilla	Vanilla oleoresin	Base

43.	Wintergreen	Gaultheria procumbens	Top
44.	Yarrow	Achillea millejolium	Middle
45.	Ylang-ylang	Cananga odorata	Middle/base

How to Recognize Quality Essential Oils

Now, it's important to point out that one brand of essential oil isn't going to be identical to another. As with many other medicinal products, there are cheap versions and there are more expensive options. Until now, you may have been wondering why you should even bother using an expensive oil if a cheaper one's just as readily available. Well, the answer is quite simple: Not all essential oils are created with the same purity in mind.

In fact, many of the cheaper versions are not 100% organic, and they may even contain filler or synthetic ingredients that can actually be *harmful* to your health. How, then, do you know if you're buying an authentic essential oil? Fortunately, I've got a few tips that you can use to buy your first batch of oils—take a look:

- **Check the bottle:** The most significant thing to look out for when you're buying essential oils is the color of the bottle. Truly, essential oils must always be in a tightly sealed dark glass bottle. This is because light exposure and heat can easily degrade the quality of the oil, which then also breaks down the aromatic compounds. Additionally, the chemical compounds in essential oils are extremely volatile and don't mix well with plastic. A word of advice here? Never buy an essential oil in a plastic bottle, no matter how convincing the label may be. Furthermore, most quality oils will come with an orifice reduction; a plastic fitting in the bottle's opening that helps regulate the amount of oil that drops out. This fitting ensures that the oil comes out one drop at a time. I recommend always looking for a bottle with this component, as it will help you measure out your oil accurately in the blending recipes.

- **Study the label:** Quality oils will clearly state the Latin name of the plant used to create the oil. For instance, lavender oil won't be labeled as such—instead, it will be labeled "Lavandula angustifolia" based on the *type of lavender plant* it comes from. In some instances, plant parts are also used, and these should also be highlighted. An example of this is the mention of "twig and leaf" commonly found on niaouli.

- **Check the source:** For the most part, quality oils will always mention the country the original plant was sourced from. A typical example of this is "Australian tea tree oil." However, the name of the country isn't always going to be listed in the name, in which case, it should always be mentioned on the bottle somewhere. If there's no mention of a country, look out for a lot number that will be written as "lot#." You can then check that number if you're unsure about the authenticity of a certain oil.

- **Compare prices:** There are very cheap essential oils out there which often make people think it's easy to stock up on a whole bunch. However, the low-priced variations should be carefully checked before you opt for them. In particular, always take a look at whether the bottle has the "100% organic" marker.

- **Avoid labels that are listed as "fragrance oil":** Simply put, essential oils shouldn't be labeled as fragrance oils. This is because, unlike essential oils, fragrance oils are *not* natural and contain many synthetic ingredients. If you're going to use your essential oils for aromatherapeutic purposes, you should definitely avoid fragrance oils.

Alright, now that you have a clearer understanding of what essential oils are, how they're made, and how they work, it's time to move on to some safety considerations for creating essential oil blends. Indeed, since these oils can be quite volatile if not mixed correctly, the next chapter is going to be quite an important read before you start mixing!

Chapter 2:

Safety Considerations and Precautions to Know Before You Create Your First Blend

Essential oils can be used as a part of your first aid kit as well. They can reduce pain, fight infections, and promote healing. –Amy Leigh Mercree

Despite being popular on the natural remedy scene, essential oils, if misused, can cause a series of adverse effects. Furthermore, as with most medications, they need to be stored correctly when not in use. On that note, this chapter is going to delve into the safety aspects of using and storing your pure essential oils, as well as the blends you're going to create.

Additionally, I'm going to answer two critical questions here: First, "Can you be allergic to essential oils?" and second, "What side effects go along with using essential oils and homemade blends?" Trust me, having the answers to these questions is going to help you make smart, safe choices with your oils from the very beginning.

How Safe Are Essential Oils for Different Demographics?

As you'll learn throughout this guide, there are numerous benefits to using essential oils. With the right blends in hand, you'll have a healthy way of dealing with stress and headaches, not to mention an aid in reducing inflammation and even improving your sleep patterns. However, does this mean that everyone in the household can use or be exposed to essential oils? Let's get into it:

- **The elderly:** Some experts recommend that elderly adults only use essential oils in a diffuser for between 15–60 minutes at a time. This is because longer exposure in a single session may cause side effects such as elevated blood pressure or heart rate. That being said, essential oils, when used in these shorter bursts, are excellent for relieving depression, decreasing anxiety, and even assisting the elderly in managing dementia. If you fall in this category and suffer from the symptoms of dementia and Alzheimer's, I recommend you speak to your practitioner about using oils such as lavender, rosemary, lemon, bergamot, ylang-ylang, ginger, and peppermint, which are all great for boosting mental capacity and improving the overall sleep quality.

- **Children**: Caution should definitely be taken when using essential oils on children. This is mostly because children have thinner skin that's much more sensitive than adults. Johns Hopkins recommends that all essential oils used on children should be diluted between 0.5–2.5% and should be avoided altogether for children under six years of age. Keep in mind that some oils such as peppermint and eucalyptus are stronger, and as such, less than half a teaspoon can lead to severe poisoning in a small child. Essential oils should also not be added to diffusers around infants younger than six months. For older children, opt to use milder oils such as sweet orange, cedarwood, or ginger. Furthermore, don't let the diffuser run for longer than an hour, and place it in a spot where it doesn't spray directly on the children. You can also speak to your pediatrician about the best oils to use.

- **Pets:** While it's true that many essential oils boast pest-repellent properties such as deterring flies and mosquitoes, it's never a good idea to spray these oils directly on their bodies. Whether ingesting or inhaling, essential oils can be harmful to both cats and dogs. If you're diffusing oils, it's best to keep your pets out of the room until you're done. Be especially cautious with high-phenol oils such as eucalyptus, clove, oregano, and wintergreen.

- **Pregnant women:** While oils such as peppermint are great for easing pregnancy symptoms, it's crucial to talk to your doctor before applying them. This is because preexisting conditions you may have can play a role in creating dangerous side effects. Also, never ingest oils—always opt to diffuse them.

- **People with respiratory conditions:** Whether or not you should use oils if you have a respiratory condition depends largely on the severity of your illness. Keep in mind that essential oils such as eucalyptus, tea tree, and peppermint can help to clear blocked airways and instantly promote healthy breathing. Of course, it's a good idea to discuss your respiratory issue and your desire to use a more natural approach with your practitioner.

Symptoms of Toxicity to Be Aware Of

It's important to note that essential oils are quickly absorbed into the skin. Same god for if they're accidentally ingested. In either case, symptoms of toxicity can appear anywhere between 30 minutes and four hours later. With a high chance of poisoning by way of either absorption method, look out for the following prominent symptoms:

- shallow breathing as well as shortness of breath
- persistent coughing or wheezing
- nausea or vomiting
- skin irritation in the form of rashes, blistering, or hives
- seizures (these are also possible in instances of large ingestion)

Since children and pets are particularly at risk, it's essential to seek medical assistance immediately after you suspect ingestion has occurred. In Chapter 3, we'll take a more extensive look at the best storage tips to implement in order to avoid accidental ingestion.

Side Effects to Be Familiar With

Fortunately, the only real side effects of essential oils are the allergic reactions that some individuals may experience from the oil or the blend. Indeed, very few essential oils actually have severe side effects such as narcotic, cancerogenic, hepatotoxic, and nephrotoxic characteristics. Indeed, in most instances, an allergic reaction or side effect actually stems from the incorrect use of a particular essential oil.

How to Tell if You're Allergic to Essential Oils

Despite its organic properties, it's possible to be allergic to a particular essential oil. Usually, an allergic reaction occurs when your immune system has an adverse reaction to an allergen in the oil or medicine. When this happens, the adverse allergen triggers your immune system to start creating antibodies, which in turn produce natural chemicals to try and expel the allergen. This allergy shows itself in the following ways:

- **Hives:** Raised red bumps or welts that itch.
- **Contact dermatitis:** A red, itchy rash that develops when your skin is exposed to an oil you're allergic to. The rash can develop into bumps, blisters, or cracked skin.
- **Phototoxic reactions:** These occur when the oil is exposed to UV rays and causes blistering or burning on the skin.
- **Nasal irritation:** This includes congestion, a runny nose, or even sneezing.
- **Eye irritation:** This can occur when you accidentally touch your eyes while using an oil, leading to burning and redness.

How to Treat an Essential Oil Allergy Reaction

Usually, you won't know that you're allergic to a particular essential oil or blend until you actually start working with it. And then, when you identify one of the above symptoms, it's important to stop using that oil or blend *immediately*. Fortunately, most essential oil-based allergic reactions can be successfully treated at home. Here are a few tips to use when you develop an adverse reaction:

- **Skin irritation:** Wash the affected skin with a mixture of cool water and mild soap. Don't scrub the skin—instead, dab and rinse.

- **Burning:** If you're experiencing a burning sensation, apply a cool, wet compress until the skin feels cooler.

- **Rash:** Apply a mild hydrocortisone cream to the burning area or rash to not only relieve the itching but also soothe any burning.

- **Eye care:** If you have accidentally splashed some essential oils in your eyes, rinse them with cool water a few times. Then, use a soft towel to dab your eyes rather than rubbing them, as rubbing may spread the oil further into your eyes. In this instance, you should seek medical advice, as your doctor may want to check for any damage behind the eyelid.

- Other instances that may require medical advice include the following:

    - **Anaphylaxis:** An allergic reaction that results in a swollen throat which will in turn lead to trouble breathing.

    - **Ingestion:** This occurs after oils have been ingested. Don't induce vomiting unless prompted to do so by an emergency responder.

Top Safety Precautions to Consider

To keep yourself and everyone in your home safe when you're using essential oils, there are several safety precautions you can follow. The following list contains the most significant ones, so feel free to peruse it:

1. **Use quality oils:** Always use quality essential oils with 100% organic ingredients. Opt for a reputable name brand that has a track record of quality products. Always read the labels of your oils and pay special attention to both the manufacturer and the medical recommendations.

2. **Check expiration dates:** Check the expiration dates of all oils you purchase. Be sure to use them within that time frame. As a rule of thumb, don't keep oils longer than three years. Label the oils that you create so that you can keep track of the expiration date.

3. **Use oils for their intended purposes:** For instance, avoid applying citrus oils topically if you're going out in the sun, as these will aggravate UV exposure.

4. **Never ingest oils:** While some manufacturers may report that their oils are safe for ingestion, keep in mind that it only takes one wrong dose or ingredient to make you violently ill. Therefore, I recommend avoiding this situation altogether by *never* ingesting any of the oils you purchase or blends you make. This includes not putting oils in your nose to clear congestion.

5. **Always speak to your medical practitioner:** If you're using your oils in conjunction with chronic medications, always discuss your intentions with your doctor. Ask them for trusted brands that have little side effects but maximum results.

6. **Don't go overboard:** You may want to add essential oils into every aspect of your life, which, in and of itself, is not a bad thing. However, incorrect dilutions may lead to a bad reaction. So, always use your oils as directed and *only* for the prescribed amount of time in your diffuser.

7. **Ensure safe storage:** Always store oils correctly to keep them out of reach of children and pets. I recommend a high-up cupboard with a child lock. The next chapter is going to provide a few more ideas here, so stay tuned!

8. **Clear up a spill immediately:** Be sure to clear up any accidental spills while you're creating your blends. Also, wash or store any tools such as droppers and spoons so that they don't pose a risk.

9. **Always diffuse in well-ventilated areas:** When it comes to diffusing your oils, always opt to place your diffuser in a well-ventilated space. A good rule of thumb is that if you can smell the oil from the diffuser, you're at risk of irritating your respiratory system. Ultimately, oils don't have to be strong to be effective. Additionally, diffusers also don't have to be on for the whole day or night in order for you to get the effect you want. In fact, exceeding the time your diffuser is on with oils can cause stress on your nervous system. Honestly, less is always more when it comes to essential oils.

10. **Dilute your oils:** If you're going to use your oils topically, never apply them directly to your skin. Instead, be sure to dilute them with quality carrier oils to safeguard your skin from irritation.

11. **Wash your hands:** Always wash your hands after you have created a blend. This is because any oils spilled on your hands can easily be transferred to your eyes, mouth, or even the inside of your ears if you touch those areas with oil on your hands. This could then lead to an adverse reaction.

12. **Keep oils away from heat:** All essential oils are highly flammable. This means that they should never be stored or used near fireplaces, lit cigarettes, candles, or gas stoves. Try to create a dedicated workstation where you can blend oils in a cool, well-ventilated space.

As you're gathering your essential oils, it's important to familiarize yourself with their ingredients, potential side effects, and the knowledge of what to do in case of an allergic reaction. Some good news here is that if you're allergic to one specific type of oil, you can easily substitute it for another that can be used for the same application.

Keep in mind that if you're not comfortable using any oils or blends on your skin, you can always just use them in a diffuser and enjoy the aroma in your living space. Once you're comfortable with your ingredients, it's time to move on to learning about the equipment, applications, and storage. So, keep reading as we dive into these aspects in Chapter 3!

Chapter 3:

Getting Started: Equipment, Applications, Blending, and Storage

Aromatherapy is a caring, hands-on therapy which seeks to induce relaxation, to increase energy, to reduce the effects of stress and to restore lost balance to mind, body, and soul. –Robert Tisserand

Alright, now that you have a better understanding of the safety precautions to consider, it's time to move on to the fun part of your essential oil journey, and by that, I mean actually getting started! Indeed, this chapter is going to dive deep into the most common oils to add to your starter kit, as well as the equipment you'll need to safely create your dream blends. Furthermore, we're going to look at some of the top applications and the general rules for blending your oils. Last but not least, we're going to cover storage and shelf life considerations, ensuring that you can keep your essential oils safe from little hands and paws— and that you use them before they deteriorate!

Top Essential Oils for Your Starter Kit

Now, if you've never bought an essential oil in your life, it can be challenging to find the first few to start your collection with. Of course, this usually depends on what you want the oil for and the types of blends you want to create. As such, I always recommend deciding on what exactly you want to use the oil *for*. Will it be for medicinal purposes? Cleaning around the house? For use in your diffuser?

Your purpose will generally determine the first few oils you should be adding to your collection. However, if you're still deciding, you may just find my starter kit list below quite useful. This list is made up of the most common oils used in general applications, as well as a few that are great for blending. Have a look:

1. **Lavender oil:** No essential oil collection will be complete without a bottle or two of lavender. Why? Because it's simply one of the most versatile essential oils. You can blend it with so many other oils, it has a relaxing and soothing aroma, and it has wonderful antibacterial properties. Then, of course, there are its amazing insect-repelling properties, which you can read all about in Chapter 6.

2. **Tea tree oil:** This gem of an oil is a personal favorite of just about every essential oil user. It's amazing for taking the sting out of a sunburn while at the same being tough on germs. It's also a great way to disinfect kitchen and bathroom surfaces.

3. **Peppermint oil:** Well-known for its refreshing aroma, peppermint oil is a great blending companion and supports respiratory issues. Additionally, it's also excellent for soothing minor aches and even adding to your bath water.

4. **Eucalyptus globulus oil:** Another oil that sits high on everyone's favorite oil list is eucalyptus. Not only does it instantly improve the energy in your space, but it also works wonders when it comes to nasal congestion. Lastly, just like tea tree oil, eucalyptus is an amazing disinfectant.

5. **Chamomile oil:** If you're familiar with the benefits of chamomile tea, you'll be delighted to learn that the oil derived from the same plant is equally great for promoting general well-being. Not only does chamomile calm a worried mind, but it also encourages peaceful sleep.

6. **Frankincense oil:** This famous oil has been around for thousands of years and is commonly used for boosting immunity. It's commonly used in the cooler months when immunity is low and common illnesses are prevalent.

7. **Lemon oil:** You'll find traces of this oil in a wide range of commercial cleaning products and toiletries. So, chances are you've been using it around your home a lot longer than you realize! With a light and zesty fragrance, it's amazing for skincare. It's also an easy oil to blend with others.

8. **Cinnamon oil:** Reputed to be one of civilization's oldest oils, cinnamon oil has antiseptic and antibacterial properties which make it a must-have in every medicine cabinet. Furthermore, it's also good for spraying in corners or the backs of cupboards where you may have spotted a rodent.

9. **Rosemary oil:** Known as a stimulant, rosemary oil has been known to be used to boost immunity and calm your nervous system. It can also decrease high levels of cortisol, the stress hormone that often leads to elevated anxiety. Rosemary oil has also become a firm favorite among those looking to boost hair and nail growth.

10. **Sweet orange oil:** If you enjoy the smell of freshly peeled orange, then this oil is the right mood booster for you. In addition to soothing digestion and calming minor aches, sweet orange oil is one of the top surface disinfectants. Its citrusy smell is well known for deterring all types of insects.

11. **Lemongrass oil:** Whether you're looking for a powerful bug repellent or simply an antifungal solution to dandruff, lemongrass oil is your one-stop solution. Its cheerful scent makes it a top choice for adding to your diffuser.

12. **Clary sage oil:** As another oil that's been used since ancient Egyptian times, clary sage is commonly used for its antidepressant properties. And when combined with lavender and marjoram, it can make the perfect massage treatment for menstrual cramping.

Chapter 8 will feature an extensive index list of the most common ailments and the essential oils that can be used to treat them.

Equipment Needed to Blend Your Oils

Okay, so the next step on your journey is going to be acquiring the right equipment and tools you'll need to start mixing and using your oils. Right off the bat, you have two main options to consider: Option one is buying each piece of equipment individually, and option two is buying a ready-packed beginner kit. In some instances, starting with one of these kits is cheaper. Plus, you can always add to your kit as you go along, depending on what you're going to be using your oils for. But feel free to start from scratch, of course!

Either way, to get started, here are some tools and pieces of equipment you'll need to consider:

1. **Anything you need for a dedicated workspace:** Whether you're going to create many different blends, or just a few to use around your home, I recommend finding a dedicated workspace. This will not only help you stay organized but will prevent accidental spills or ingestions if you're working on the coffee table. So, get yourself a dedicated desk or table, maybe some small sorting baskets, and, of course, some paper and a pen never hurt for keeping track of your oils, measurements, etc.

2. **Bottle and jars:** No matter how tempted you are to buy quirky little clear bottles, steer clear from any that aren't green, amber, or blue. Furthermore, start with smaller bottles such as 5ml, 10ml, or 30ml. Keep in mind that bottles with dripolators (the plastic piece that fits into a bottle to regulate flow to a drop) are better for essential oils than dropper heads. The bottles will depend on what you're going to make, though, so decide on this before you go out and buy hundreds of the same type of bottles. On top of that, oil blends will require different bottles than those used for cremes, butter, or balms. So, if you're going

to use plastic containers for the creams, be sure to opt for PET bottles, or else the essential oils will degrade the plastic. I prefer glass bottles and jars as they can be reused, unlike plastic which ends up in landfills and harms the environment.

3. **Glass mixing equipment:** You're going to have to set a few glass mixing bowls and beakers aside for mixing. Don't use the ones from your baking cupboard, though, as there's always the risk of cross-contamination. Typically, a few glass beakers and one or two bowls will be all you need to mix oils and creams in. If you live in the US, discount and dollar stores are the perfect places to find these beakers at a very affordable price. I also recommend using glass or metal stirring rods as opposed to plastic. Once again, plastic is bad for the environment and also retains odors which contributes to cross-contamination.

4. **Labels:** You will need labels to mark the blends you're creating. Of course, how professional-looking your labels are depends on what you're making the oils for. If you're making the oils for yourself, you might not mind plain labels on which you can jot down the ingredients and the date blended. If you're making a blend as a gift for someone, however, it's a good idea to opt for smudge-free labels.

5. **A quality scale:** Your blending journey will benefit from a quality scale and a glass measuring jug. You'll want to have equipment that can give you accurate measurements whether you're measuring out oil or cream.

6. **Perfume testing strips:** While you're technically not creating perfume, these strips are an excellent way to test the aromatics of your blend. These are especially handy in the early days when you're still new to the blending process and not sure if you've done it correctly.

7. **Sundries:** You should also opt for a few sundries such as tweezers, cotton swabs, and 70% isopropyl alcohol for cleaning your tools, mixing bowls, and work surface. You may also want to have a pair of gloves in your work kit in case you're creating

a blend for someone else that contains an ingredient that irritates your skin.

Top Applications of Common Essential Oils

If you speak to people who regularly use essential oils, you'll soon realize that there's no one-size-fits-all approach when it comes to the best ways to apply or blend oils. Since not all oils are the same, you'll find that some are better suited for specific applications. The most common applications include the following:

- **Topical applications:** One of the more common application methods involves creating a blend that can be applied topically. This, then, will usually involve massaging or rubbing the oil blend onto the skin. In this instance, you can rub the oil blend directly onto your skin or, if you prefer, you can add it to a compatible cream, lotion, or skin butter. The best essential oils to use for topical application are as follows:

    - lavender
    - tea tree
    - ylang-ylang
    - rosehip
    - geranium

- **Diffusers:** Typically, a diffuser is a device that distributes essential oils into the air of the room it's in. Diffusers can be made from a range of materials such as ceramic, ultrasonic, candle, and even reed. It's important to follow the manufacturer guidelines of your specific diffuser type. Keep in mind, too, that diffusers are an effective alternative for applying oils directly to your skin or inhaling them. Also, the size of your diffuser will determine the amount of oil you need to add. Here are a few examples of the most common oils to use in a diffuser:

- lavender to aid in sleeping
- eucalyptus for easy breathing
- jasmine for boosting your mood
- ginger to treat nausea

- **Steam inhalers:** Using the steam inhalation method is quite popular among people with cold and flu symptoms or even to clear chest congestion. Here's how you can do this:

    - Add a few drops of essential oil to a bowl of hot water. Consider using an oil such as eucalyptus because of its congestion-clearing properties.
    - Place a towel over your head and be sure to cover the bowl as well. (Essentially, what you're doing is forming a tent over both your head and the bowl.)
    - Close your eyes and deeply inhale this steam mixture for a few minutes. Take deep breaths to ensure that you get the mixture deep into your chest.
    - Repeat this a few times throughout the day or at times when you feel overly congested.

- **Dry inhalation:** For this application, you'll only need some type of dry material such as a piece of fabric or cotton swab. All you need to do is as follows:

    - Add a few drops of your favorite essential oils to the material.
    - Hold the material to your nose and allow the scent of the oil to disperse naturally.

- You can add these cotton swabs to your pillowcase, shirt pocket, or even your car vents.

- Chamomile, peppermint, and lavender are firm favorites for this method.

- **Steam baths:** Essential oils are particularly useful in the bath or shower. You can either add a few drops of your favorite oils to your body wash, shampoo, or even conditioner. Additionally, you can also add a few drops to your shower walls as this will enable you to inhale the oil as a steam. Now, if you want to add some oil to your bath water, remember to dilute it with a carrier or base oil. You can also add a few drops to the bubble bath or mix the oil with bicarbonate of soda and Epsom salt to create a salt bath. In Chapter 5, we'll be going over some ideal blends for this exact purpose, so keep an eye out for those!

- **Mist sprays:** Using essential oils in a spritzer bottle is a wonderfully easy way to get essential oil into the air in your space without a diffuser. All it takes is a few drops of oil mixed with purified or distilled water. Just be sure to give the bottle a good shake before you spray. Also, keep animals and small children out of the room you're spraying in. These are the best oils for sprays:

    - peppermint to deter pests

    - lavender to help you sleep

    - chamomile to help you relax

Blending and Dilution Guidelines

To create safe and effective oils, it's important to adhere to a few blending and dilution guidelines. This will not only help you prevent potential skin irritation but also make your bottle of essential oil last longer. Some critical guidelines for this subject will be discussed below.

Handy Blending Chart

The chart below is a simple reference guide for the basic ratios required to make some mild essential oil blends. This should help you get an idea of the amount of essential oil versus the carrier oil required.

The first column refers to a percentage that applies to instances where a recipe blend requires you to add a certain percentage of essential oil to a cream, lotion, or other substance that you're working with.

Percent of Essential Oil Required	Essential Oil Quantity	Carrier Oil Quantity
0.5%	<ul><li>1 drop</li><li>2 drops</li><li>10 drops</li></ul>	<ul><li>2 tsp</li><li>1 tbsp</li><li>100ml</li></ul>
1%	<ul><li>2 drops</li><li>4 drops</li><li>20 drops</li></ul>	<ul><li>2 tsp</li><li>1 tbsp</li><li>100ml</li></ul>
2%	<ul><li>4 drops</li><li>8 drops</li><li>40 drops</li></ul>	<ul><li>2 tsp</li><li>1 tbsp</li><li>100ml</li></ul>
3%	<ul><li>6 drops</li><li>12 drops</li><li>60 drops</li></ul>	<ul><li>2 tsp</li><li>1 tbsp</li><li>100ml</li></ul>

Rules for Blending Essential Oils

So, as you're preparing to blend your different essential oils, there are a few rules to stick with. Here, in particular, are the most significant ones to be aware of:

- Plan your blend and review the ingredients you want to use before you start mixing.

- A general rule of thumb is to avoid exceeding the 3% dilution rate for the mixture, as this will ensure it remains effective.

- Let your blend stand for 48 hours before using it to ensure it mixes correctly.

- Once again, essential oils should never be consumed orally or applied directly to your skin.

Blending Classifications

Essential oil blends are typically divided into four different classifications. These classifications highlight the order in which they should be added to the blend to ensure it mixes correctly.

1. **The Personifier:** Oils in this category should be added to the blend first because they typically have the strongest fragrances. Furthermore, their dominant properties also make them perfect for therapeutic purposes. These oils should make up 1–5% of your blend. A few of the more common oils in this category include these:

    - clove
    - mandarin
    - peppermint
    - clary sage

- ylang-ylang

2. **The Enhancer:** These oils should be the most predominant in the blend. They should also emphasize the properties of the other oils you're adding. Their fragrance is milder than a Personifier and should make up about 50–80% of the blend. A few examples of these include the following:

    - eucalyptus
    - lavender
    - basil
    - lemon
    - cedarwood

3. **The Equalizer:** When creating your blend, you want your oils to create a balance, as this will affect their efficacy. They should also not exceed 10–15% of the overall mixture. The most common of these include the following:

    - tea tree
    - sandalwood
    - basil
    - ginger

4. **The Modifier:** Oils in this category add overall harmony to the blend. They shouldn't exceed 5–8% of the blend. A few examples of these oils include the following:

    - eucalyptus
    - lemon
    - cardamom

- coriander
- rose

Safe Dilution Guidelines

Now, the strength and ratio of your blend should be made with the age and application in mind. For instance, children and older adults will need a milder blend. Here are a few tips to help you safely dilute your oils:

- **Adults:** On average, 2–3% is a safe dilution ratio for overall topical application in adults. This usually means that you can use about 10–15 drops of essential oil for every 1 ounce (30 ml) of carrier oil. These are the most recommended carrier oils for topical applications:
    - almond oil
    - grapeseed oil
    - coconut oil
- **Children and the elderly:** As I mentioned in the previous chapter, essential oils can be too harsh for older people and children alike. However, if your medical practitioner has given you the go-ahead, opt for a dilution ratio of 1% or less. Usually, this amounts to about 5 drops of essential oil for every 1 ounce (30ml) of carrier oil.
- **Babies and infants:** As with children and the elderly, extreme care should be given to any essential oil use. In particular, a dilution ratio of 0.2–0.5% is the maximum you should use for babies between 3–24 months. This equates to 1–3 drops of essential oil for 1 ounce (30ml) of carrier oil.

Measurement Conversion Table

When I started on my essential oil journey, I often found it challenging to find the correct measurements for my blends. Some recipes would call for drops, while others would have the ingredients listed in ounces. And if you prefer to have measurements in the metric system, you may find yourself having to do your own conversions as I often did!

This is frustrating, to say the least. However, it's with this frustration in mind that I decided to make my own measurement conversion table that I hope will come in handy for you too!

Drop Conversions	Milliliters/Ounces
20 drops	1ml
75 drops	3.75ml
100 drops	5ml
150 drops	7.5ml
200 drops	10ml
300 drops	15ml
600 drops	30ml
12.5 drops	⅛ tsp
25 drops	¼ tsp
50 drops	½ tsp
75 drops	¾ tsp

100 drops	1 tsp
300 drops	1 tbsp
600 drops	1 ounce
1.200 drops	2 ounces
2.400 drops	4 ounces
3.600 drops	6 ounces
4.800 drops	8 ounces

Storage Tips to Keep in Mind

Let me share with you two solid reasons as to why essential oils should be stored correctly. The first has to do with oxidation, and the other with general safety. Let's dig into these a little deeper.

First of all, oxidation happens when the oil is exposed to excessive oxygen. Typically, this happens as a result of changes in the molecular bonds in the oil. In short, cells in the oxygen bonds are converted into carbon bonds, which then causes the general composition of the oil to change, affecting its strength and overall effectiveness. Once this happens, we enter the second reason—general safety. Indeed, it becomes difficult to determine the safety levels of the oils, especially since factors such as initial quality and storage also contribute to the process.

That said, there are a few tips to consider when you're planning to store your oils and blends. These are as follows:

- **Make sure lids are always on tight:** The lid on your bottle should always be on tight. This will prevent air and water from getting inside the bottle, and it will also reduce oxidation. On top of those reasons, tight lids will also keep bacteria from getting into the bottle and prevent evaporation.

- **Keep the plastic fitment on:** If you're planning to make a large quantity of an essential oil blend, you may be tempted to remove the plastic fitment that's usually found on the bottle. But resist! Why? Because this fitment doesn't only help to keep oil from spilling out, but it also keeps moisture and air from entering the bottle. So, yes, I suggest keeping the plastic fitment on, no matter how annoyed you may be with the oil coming out one drop at a time.

- **Avoid direct sunlight and heat:** As I've mentioned previously, direct sunlight and heat can significantly affect the quality of your essential oil. Generally, too much heat can cause the oil to evaporate faster which, in turn, makes it less effective. In short, exposure to the sun deteriorates the properties of your oil.

- **Opt for a cool, dark place:** Whether you're using oils in your business or for personal reasons, you may be tempted to display them on a shelf in the open. However, try to avoid this for long periods, as oil bottles must be kept in a cool, dark place away from heat and direct sunlight. On that note, it's always a good idea to place your oils in a cupboard that's out of reach of children or wandering pets. If you're opting for a shelf, make sure it's high enough to prevent children from reaching it.

- **Store while you're traveling:** If you're like me, you may want to take your oils with you wherever you go especially if you're using them for therapeutic purposes or you're going on holiday. In this instance, look for a specially designed carrying case to keep your oils upright and out of the sun.

Shelf Life Considerations

In addition to considering storage tips, it's also important to discuss the shelf life considerations that go along with safe essential oil usage.

Indeed, when you're setting out to buy your first bunch of oils, you may be wondering whether they expire and what can be done to extend their normal shelf life. Well, the next section is going to answer both of these questions and also highlight the best way to "dispose" of older oils.

Do Essential Oils Expire?

Typically, it's not the age of an oil that makes it less useful—rather, it's the amount of oxidation it has been exposed to. For instance, the suggested lifespan of a particular oil may be five years. However, if the oil isn't stored correctly, or the bottle is continuously left open while you're blending, chances are the quality of the oil will degrade a lot faster.

So, while an essential oil doesn't "go bad" in the way a fruit or a veggie would, it's hard to establish how safe they are after their suggested lifespan. In particular, experts advise against inhaling or applying oils to your skin if they are past their use-by date.

Simple Ways to Extend the Shelf Life of Essential Oils

Since quality essential oils can be quite pricey, it's only natural to want to extend their shelf life for as long as possible. On that note, there are a few tips that you can implement to extend the shelf life of your oils and blends. These are listed as follows:

- **Buy as you need:** Instead, try to top up your stock, as this is better than ending up with several bottles that aren't fresh in two years.

- **Keep them sealed:** Only open the bottles when you're going to use them. There's no need to open them to sniff their fragrance on the day you buy them. And once opened, make sure they don't remain open for too long. Use what you need and seal the bottle quickly and tightly.

- **Store the oils in dark amber bottles:** Never transfer your oils to lighter bottles or other containers. Instead, keep them in the dark bottles they were in when you bought them. Your blends should also be in dark bottles to eliminate light exposure.

- **Avoid direct light and heat:** It's a good idea to store your bottles in a dark cupboard where they're not only out of reach of little hands but also away from heat and light.

- **Store blends in smaller bottles:** Storing your blends correctly is equally as important as keeping your store-bought variants safe. A simple way to increase the shelf life of your homemade blends is to put them in smaller bottles. In fact, this will prevent oxygen from being trapped in the bottle when it's opened, and at the same time, it will delay the whole oxidation process.

Shelf Life of Common Essential Oils

The average shelf life of the more common essential oils ranges between two to five years if they have been sealed correctly and stored in a cool, dark place. They should also be in dark bottles and kept out of direct light and away from heat. A few oils, such as sandalwood, vetiver, and patchouli can even last for six to eight years under the right conditions.

Below, I've compiled a handy table to help you keep track of your oils. I recommend writing the date bought or blended on all bottles to be sure your oils are also safe and fresh.

General Shelf Life	Essential Oils
1–2 years	- Lime
	- Lemon
	- Tangerine
2–3 years	- Tea tree
	- Lemongrass

3–4 years	- Copaiba - Black pepper - Bergamot - Cypress - Spearmint - Frankincense - Melissa - Rosemary - Helichrysum - Lavender - Eucalyptus - Clary sage - Cinnamon bark - Cardamon - Myrrh - Vanilla oleoresin
4–5 years	- Peppermint - Cedarwood - Ylang-ylang - Blue tansy

6–8 years	- Wintergreen - Vetiver - Sandalwood - Patchouli

What to Do With "Expired" Essential Oils

While it's true that essential oils don't expire in the true sense of the word, it's important to point out that they can still oxidize to the point where they're no longer suitable for medicinal purposes. Now, if you suspect that some of your oils are past their prime, the good news is that you don't have to throw them away. Just because you can't use them on your skin doesn't mean they're completely useless. Consider these options:

- **Add them to a diffuser:** The general rule of thumb is that an essential oil is still good to be used in a diffuser if you can still enjoy the scent. That, of course, means the scent shouldn't be dull or stale. In these instances, you can easily use the oil in your diffuser to freshen the air in your home.

- **Place a few drops in the laundry:** You can also use the "expired" oils to keep your clothes and sheets smelling fresh. Simply add a drop or two to your laundry. The rule here is to avoid applying the oils directly to the fabric, though, as this can lead to staining. I usually add a few drops to my washing machine while washing bedding or curtains. Lavender, peppermint, or lemon are especially great.

- **Use them as part of your cleaning routine:** Essential oils that are not that fresh can still be used to clean everything from windows to fridges. Just dilute them and add them to a spray bottle. From there, go ahead and spritz on surfaces that can do with cleaning and a fresh fragrance. Lemon is wonderful for kitchen surfaces.

Well, this has been quite a comprehensive chapter. Truly, though, understanding things like blend ratios and safe storage is an absolutely crucial step in creating the foundation of your essential oil journey.

Moving on, the next chapter is going to take an in-depth look at advanced blending techniques best suited for beginners. Additionally, I'm going to share a few unconventional essential oils that are worth trying out—so keep reading for more on these!

Chapter 4:

Advanced Blending Techniques

I mix all different oils—my bathroom at home is littered with oils; I'm really into natural beauty and natural healing. Peppermint is really good if you put it on your stomach for a tummy ache; lavender is kind of all-purpose—I think everyone should carry it. –Liz Goldwyn

Blending your essential oils is about a lot more than simply mixing your favorite oils and hoping for an effective blend. For starters, you'll need to decide what you want the blend to do and how you're going to apply it. And before you start blending, you'll also need to have an idea of your reaction to never-before-used oils to ensure you steer clear of any allergic reactions.

So, to help you kick off your blending adventure, this chapter is going to walk you through a few techniques to consider and a few unconventional oils to add to your collection. I'll also be sharing some information on synergy oil blends and why they're worth looking into. Now, let's get moving!

Advanced Blending Techniques

Essentially, there are three top ways to group your blending techniques. These are:

Blending by Effect

So, this first technique refers to creating blends that offer a specific effect or purpose. That essentially means that the oils you're combining should all contribute to the overall expectation. For instance, if you want a relaxing blend that you can add to your diffuser just before bed, then it makes sense to avoid including any oils that are energizing.

By that rationale, if you want to create a blend that you're going to use as a cleaning agent, you will want to combine oils with superior cleaning properties. Typically, creating a blend for a specific effect or purpose is often divided into four sections, highlighted in the table below.

General Purpose	Best Oils to Blend Together
Energizing (These blends are primarily used to kick-start your day or give you a boost of energy when you need it most)	- Basil - Rosemary - Tea tree - Pine needle - Lemon - Grapefruit - Citronella - Coriander - Spearmint - Eucalyptus - Clove - Cypress - Lime
Relaxing	- Lavender - Frankincense

(These oils can also be used to create mood-enhancing blends)	- Cedarwood
- Ylang-ylang
- Bergamot
- Geranium
- Palmarosa
- Nutmeg
- Red thyme
Cleansing (Many of the oils in this section can also be used to create blends that deter pests)	- Lemon
- Peppermint
- Sweet orange
- Citronella
- Grapefruit
- Lime
- Oregano
- Patchouli
- Juniper berry
Grounding (These blends should create a balance of fragrances that boost spirituality and enhance feelings of clarity and positivity)	- Black pepper
- Frankincense
- Sandalwood
- Chamomile

	- Spearmint
- Marjoram
- Geranium
- Bergamot
- Lavender
- Oregano

Blending by Fragrance

Some essential oils are well known for having amazing scents, while others can be quite overpowering. As such, it's important to mix oils in similar fragrance groups to avoid creating a blend that has an overpowering scent, which can lead to allergies or even add to a headache you're trying to pacify.

While you can divide your essential oils into many different fragrance categories, I recommend simplifying the process by focusing on five fundamental groups. This is because oils based in the same fragrance group will generally blend well together and minimize the chances of contrasting or overbearing fragrances. Furthermore, blending by fragrance is a good technique to opt for if you just want to use blends for the sake of adding fragrances to your home. The five categories that serve as a good place to start are listed in the table below.

Fragrance Category	Fragrance to Blend With	Essential Oils to Blend With
Floral	Blends with spicy, woody, floral, and herbal fragrances	- Geranium
- Lavender
- Ylang-ylang

Citrus	Blends with woody, floral, spicy, and herbal fragrances	- Palmarosa
- Lemon
- Lime
- Grapefruit
- Citronella
- Bergamot
- Lemongrass
- Sweet orange
- Grapefruit
- Citronella
Spicy	Blends with woody, floral, and citrus fragrances	- Cinnamon
- Peppermint
- Coriander
- Nutmeg
- Black pepper
- Clove
Woody	Blend with citrus, floral, spicy, and herbal fragrances	- Sandalwood
- Pine needle
- Cypress
- Juniper

		• Patchouli
		• Frankincense
Herbal	Blend with spicy and woody fragrances	• Sage
		• Thyme
		• Tea tree
		• Rosemary
		• Marjoram
		• Eucalyptus
		• Chamomile
		• Basil
		• Spearmint

Blending by Note

Essential oils evaporate at varying speeds, and this means that not mixing your oils by note can result in a blend that smells different a few months after you create it. So, if you use a weaker note, the stronger oil will overpower the blend with time. As discussed in Chapter 3, top notes fade the fastest, followed by middle notes. Meanwhile, base notes last the longest. Feel free to refer back to my table in Chapter 1 for a list of different oils that fall into top, middle, and base note categories.

The 30/50/20 Blending Note Rule

If you're opting to blend by note, it's a good idea to use the 30/50/20 rule. This common rule states that your blend should be made up of 30% top note oils, 50% middle note oils, and 20% base note oils. Essentially, that means if you're creating a blend that requires 10 drops of oil in total, you should use three drops of a top note oil, five drops of a middle note, and then two drops of a base note. Without a doubt, this simple formula will help you create the most harmonious blend.

Basic Blending Tips to Consider

Once you know what you want to do with your oils, it's time to start blending. Here are a few quick steps to get you started:

- **Step 1:** Clear your workspace, open a window for ventilation, and get your bottles, tools, and oils ready.

- **Step 2:** Have your recipe at hand so you don't get confused or miss a step.

- **Step 3:** Add the required number of drops of each oil to your amber bottle. Do one oil at a time, and close the bottle before moving to the next oil. Stir the blend as you mix for it to start mixing. Don't exceed the 3% dilution rate.

- **Step 4:** Check the balance of the blend by giving it a light sniff. Keep in mind that the oil will change as the oils blend, so avoid tweaking the fragrance too much.

- **Step 5:** Close the bottle tightly and add a label. It's a good idea to add the ingredients on the label, however, if your label is too small, label your blend as "Blend 1" and then list the ingredients in your notebook for future reference.

- **Step 6:** Leave your blend to "settle" for 48 hours before using. If the blend isn't quite what you had in mind, don't waste the oil by discarding it. Instead, use it in a diffuser or refer back to Chapter 3 for tips on discarding oils you can no longer use for the intended purpose.

Unconventional Essential Oils and Blends

When you're starting out on your essential oil journey, chances are you're only going to buy a handful of what I like to call the "usual favorites." These are oils like lavender, eucalyptus, peppermint, chamomile, lemon, and basil. And they're favorites for a reason—indeed, they can be used for the most applications, and in some instances, they're also the most readily available.

Now, as great as the usual favorites are, as a beginner, you also shouldn't be afraid to explore a few other options on the market. Indeed, once you're comfortable with your collection of go-tos, why not explore the benefits of some more unusual oils? In particular, a few of my own recently discovered favorites are listed below:

- **Hinoki essential oil:** When it comes to unconventional essential oils, one of the more common is hinoki, which comes from the leaves of Japanese cypress trees. You can expect a light, woody scent with a hint of lemon from this oil, and it's excellent for adding to your diffuser when you're meditating, having a yoga session, or simply just looking to refresh your mind. Hinoki can easily be mixed with lemon and frankincense to enhance its citrusy sweetness too.

- **Cistus essential oil:** If you enjoy adding oils with floral notes to your diffuser, then the honey-like scent of cistus is a must-add to your collection. Its gentle, floral fragrance makes a great blending partner for sage, tangerine, and lemon myrtle. Made from the magenta flowered rockrose bush, this oil is perfect for creating a relaxing bath tea or making a quick linen spray.

- **Raven essential oil:** With a refreshing, minty, fragrance, this delightful oil is a combination of wintergreen, peppermint, lemon, and eucalyptus. This wonderful combination means you'll have the perfect blend for your diffuser whenever your home feels a little stuffy. To enhance its invigorating fragrance, try blending it with geranium and myrrh.

- *Xiang Mao* **essential oil:** Your first whiff of this green-citrus scent will leave you with a sense of familiarity. The reason for this is that *Xiang Mao* oil is traditionally used in most commercial air-fresheners. In addition to refreshing musty or smelly rooms, this earthy essential oil is also wonderful for creating an uplifting scent once it swirls through your diffuser. It also blends well with marjoram and nutmeg!

- **Goldenrod essential oil**: Despite its many beauty and relaxation benefits, you may be surprised to learn that this essential oil smells like licorice. It's great for mixing with sage and then adding to your skincare creams. Furthermore, rubbing it on your feet at night will ensure you're one step closer to having a restful sleep.

Synergy Blends

I've said this before, but it's important to emphasize it again: No two essentials are going to be identical. Indeed, each oil has its own unique properties that make it effective for its intended purpose. That said, some oils work better on their own while others may be more effective as part of a specialized blend. These specially mixed blends are often referred to as "synergy blends". Let's take a more in-depth look at this concept.

What Are Synergy Oils?

Based on the Greek word, "*sunergos*," the word "synergy" simply refers to the concept of working together. This concept, then, involves using the strengths of different components to create a more potent effect.

Here's a practical example: Lavender oil on its own is excellent for many ailments such as headaches. However, when correctly blended with peppermint, rosemary, marjoram, chamomile, and wintergreen, you get a much more potent blend that not only reduces tension but eases the mental stressors that caused your headache or migraine in the first place.

As you can see, the synergy mixture is more robust and effective than the lavender is on its own.

How Do Synergy Oils Work?

Simply put, synergy oils are specially designed to optimize and maximize the effect and value of each ingredient. Of course, this means they should be used with specific purposes in mind. The most common of these include the following:

- to soothe continuous pain
- to support immunity
- to promote mental clarity
- to encourage relaxation

Typically, synergy blends work better than simply applying a single oil because the components in specific oils facilitate chemical reactions in other oils that end up creating the desired effect.

Now, keep in mind that this effect can only be achieved if you mix the right oils in the exact quantities. By this, I mean that mixing lavender with peppermint oil may be more effective than simply using lavender alone. However, you still won't achieve the maximum effect that mixing the oils in the above example would provide you with.

Benefits of Using Synergy Blends

There are many benefits to using ready-made synergy oils. Here are a few of the most prominent:

- **Convenience:** Beginners find ready-made synergy blends more practical to use while they learn the art of blending the right oil mixes. It's also quicker if you need relief from a nagging ailment such as a headache or insomnia.

- **Making for more potent mixes:** Unlike regular mixed oils that often only have two or three ingredients, synergy blends are specially designed to combine the characteristics of certain oils to target a specific ailment.

- **Affordability:** Quality essential oils can be expensive especially if you're buying several bottles at once to create a synergy blend. This is another reason why beginners opt for ready-made synergy blends to treat ailments while they build their stocks to begin blending.

- **Flexibility:** As with regular blends, synergy oils can be very flexible. They can be added to creams, serums, lotions, base oils, candles, scrubs, and roll-ons. They can also be diffused for maximum results.

Buying Ready-Made Synergy Blends

Beginners often shy away from mixing their own synergy blends because the number of ingredients in each blend can seem overwhelming. Fortunately, many essential oil suppliers *do* offer a synergy blend range that you can use until you're comfortable creating your own.

If this is an option you're considering, suppliers such as New Directions Aromatics have a few top options to consider. In fact, to give you an idea of the ingredients in a typical synergy blend, the table below is going to focus on this specific supplier's offerings (New Directions Aromatics, 2024).

Name of the New Direction Synergy Blend	Ingredients	Ailments to Treat
Head Ease Synergy Blend	- Peppermint - Rosemary - Sweet basil	Directly treats mental stressors associated with various types of headaches and migraines.

	<ul><li>Wintergreen</li><li>Chamomile</li><li>Lavender</li><li>Marjoram</li><li>Frankincense</li></ul>	
Breathe Easy Synergy Blend	<ul><li>Eucalyptus</li><li>Peppermint</li><li>Cardamom</li><li>*Ravintsara*</li><li>Laurel leaf</li></ul>	Assists with clearing nasal or chest congestion as well as alleviating stress and tension symptoms.
Mental Clarity Synergy Blend	<ul><li>Grapefruit</li><li>Basil</li><li>Lemon</li><li>Bergamot</li></ul>	Excellent for assisting with mental clarity and enhancing focus needed for decisive thought.

Of course, this table only shows three examples of synergy oils. Each supplier may have different names for their in-house blends and ingredients may vary slightly. The trick, then, is to find the characteristics from specific blends that, when combined, will provide you with a more potent oil.

Many of the regular essential oil blends involve mixing two or three oils to give you a mixture you can use for basic ailments. As you grow on your essential oil journey, though, it may be a good idea to practice creating the more complex synergy blends—especially for recurring ailments like sinuses or headaches.

Tips to Effectively Use Synergy Oils

Alright, so if you're going to try out a few synergy blends to treat an ailment, there are a few tips to keep in mind to ensure that you're using them safely. A few of these are as follows:

- **Opt for quality:** As with buying individual essential oils, it's important to opt for quality synergy blends. These should be 100% pure and natural blends that have been designed by aromatherapy experts. This will ensure that the safest quantities have been used to create each blend. A supplier website should specify the ingredients used to ensure you avoid exposure to any oil that you're allergic to.

- **Make sure it's diluted:** Since synergy blends are made of a mixture of many different oils, they tend to be super concentrated. This means they should never be applied directly to the skin. The NDA (that is, New Directions Aromatics)recommendation is that each blend should be diluted between 3–5% for safe topical applications. Diffusion is also a viable option to get optimal results.

- **Always follow instructions:** No matter how long you've been using essential oils, always be sure to read and follow the instructions on the label or website. Keep in mind that some oils are light-sensitive, which means they're better suited for nighttime use. On top of that, phototoxic oils shouldn't be applied to the skin if you spend a day in the sun. Also, always avoid blends that aren't labeled.

- **Don't adjust the formula:** It's important to remember that synergy blends have been specially designed in different ratios to create a specific effect for a certain ailment. So, in short, don't alter the premixed formula. If your blend smells too strong, don't be tempted to add some lavender to make it more flowery!

Ultimately, choosing a blending technique doesn't have to be a complex process. All you have to do is decide which technique you want to start with. Opting for the note technique is often the best place for beginners, as this tends to create the most balanced blend, no matter what the application will be. Stick to the basic tips I've suggested and you'll be well on your way to becoming a blending pro before you know it!

And now, as you start perfecting your blending techniques, it's time to start creating the blends that can treat your family's ailments. That's right, in Chapter 5, we're going to be taking an extensive look at the various therapeutic benefits of using essential oils and their relevant blends. Furthermore, I'll be sharing several recipes to get your blending journey well and truly started!

Chapter 5:

Therapeutic Benefits of Essential Oils

Essential oils are the bridge that connects our physical and spiritual well-being.
–Unknown

As I've said before in this guide, essential oils have been around for what seems like, well, *forever*. And with their antibacterial and antifungal properties, it's no wonder that aromatherapy's popularity persists all the way to the present day. Indeed, since each oil has a distinct composition and a unique chemical makeup, they can be used for everything from light mood enhancement to pain relief.

However, it's important to understand which oils work best for which ailments, and how much should be applied. With that in mind, this chapter is going to offer you an in-depth look at the most common ailments that will benefit from an essential oil treatment, as well as a few of the best suggestions to make your first healing blends. Furthermore, I'm also going to share a few top tips for including essential oils in your daily self-care and overall wellness routine. After all, to experience optimum results, essential oils should be used daily!

Are Essential Oils a Suitable Alternative to Medicine?

Now, you've likely heard about all the wonderful results so many people seem to be having with their various essential oil blends. In fact, some may prefer to use their own homemade blends for ailments such as headaches, sunburn, stress, nausea, overexposure, winding down, and a host of stomach issues. This obviously begs the question—should we use essential oils as an alternative to conventional medicine?

Well, currently, the Food and Drug Administration classifies essential oils in the category of cosmetic treatments, as they don't contain the chemicals actually needed to treat and prevent disease (Farrar & Farrar, 2020). At the same time, I must also point out that a particular oil won't always have the same effect on each person. For instance, peppermint oil in capsule form may prove wonderful for *my* gut issues, but it might end up having zero effect on another person with the same symptoms.

Furthermore, you may have better results with a particular oil despite there being a bunch of others who profess to do the same thing. For instance, lavender has an amazing calming effect on me, especially at night, but chamomile may work better for you. Therefore, it's important to keep the following precautions in mind as you set out to incorporate essential oils into your daily routine:

- **Stick to the recommendations:** Always use the prescribed amount of essential oils when you're creating blends. It's also important to use the suggested amounts in all your applications to avoid overexposure.

- **Speak to your practitioner:** Don't substitute your prescribed medicine with essential oil blends without first speaking to your practitioner or a certified aromatherapist.

- **Start small:** Create a blend for the ailment you experience the most frequently. For instance, if you're consistently suffering from anxiety, it's a good idea to start with a calming blend and monitor the effects it has on you. Then, if your workblend doesn't seem to do the trick, you may want to consider a synergy blend. (Consider taking another look at the specialized blends discussed in Chapter 4.)

- **Use blends for the simple stuff:** Let's face it, you're not going to outright cure your gut health with an essential oil overnight. You can, however, use an oil for something like easing the painful effects of sunburn. And, of course, essential oils are also great for adding to your winding-down routine in the evening. Adding them to your bath water and diffuser will also help soothe your nerves and your general mood. So no, they won't work on treating major ailments, but the more you use the oils and the specialized blends you create in smaller but still meaningful areas of your life, the better your general health will be.

Most Common Ailments That Can Be Treated With Essential Oils

While essential oils are not a substitute for medicines provided by your medical practitioner, they remain a popular alternative for *minor* ailments. On top of that, they can actually play a key role in helping people reduce the amount of medications they take. For instance, if you're already taking chronic medications, you may not want to pile on the pills when you're struggling with ailments such as headaches, sunburn, nausea, and even minor aches. And as you know by now, your oils and/or blends can prove to be just the right alternative in these situations.

With a wide range of essential oils commercially available and an endless list of blends you can create in the comfort of your own home, finding the right blend for your ailment has truly never been easier. We've touched on some of these already, but here are a few of the more common ailments that can be treated with a variety of essential oil blends:

- headaches
- anxiety
- low appetite
- nausea

- sunburn

- stress relief

In addition to these, oil blends can also aid in reducing fever, boosting mood, and fighting certain infections. In Chapter 8, we'll be looking at a handy ailment index table that highlights the various essential oils you can use for different ailments. Be sure to check it out!

Recipe Blends and the Best Ways to Apply Them for the Most Common Ailments

Now that you've read about the safety precautions, types of blends you can create, and the best application methods to consider, it's time to get to the fun part—creating your own blends! As I've said, this process is not just going to involve you mixing a bunch of oils and hoping for the best. Not a chance. Instead, your mixing is going to be methodical and productive. And the best place to start? Gathering up a few potential blend recipes.

Of course, as you get ready to pursue these recipes, be sure to have a notebook handy to make notes about the quantities and types of oils you're creating. This will help you keep track of the blends that work well, and enable you to tweak the ones that aren't so effective. To help get you started, I've compiled a list below of the most common blends that work well for basic ailments.

Blend # 1: Headache Blend

I suffer from headaches quite a lot. I chalk it up to a combination of stress, heat, and humidity. And to make matters worse, I'm not a big fan of popping pills. Why? Well, because, continuously taking back pills for one thing or the other can ultimately have a detrimental effect on one's gut health.

As such, finding a more holistic approach to dealing with my headaches was one of the driving factors in my own essential oil journey. And today, I'm happy to announce that I've had a great deal of success with several different headache blends! Here's the blend I've found to be the most effective for migraines:

Ingredients

- 3 drops of peppermint oil
- 2 drops of lavender oil

Method

- Add to a diffuser and let it run for a few hours in the room you're in.
- Remember to keep small children and pets away from the area where the diffuser is.

Blend # 2: On-The-Go Headache Blend

Having a handy on-the-go blend is also great for those days when you and your diffuser aren't together. My go-to recipe for that is as follows:

Ingredients

- 4 drops of lavender oil
- 4 drops of peppermint oil
- 2 drops of rosemary oil

Method

- Place the oil in a 10ml roller ball bottle and fill it with jojoba oil. (Remember to use a dark-colored bottle.)
- Dot the blend on your forehead and temples and massage it gently into your skin.

- Be sure to wash your hands before accidentally rubbing any oil into your eyes.

Blend #3: Insect Shield

Insect bites can be very annoying, and at the same time, bug sprays can be quite costly. If you prefer a natural approach to keeping those pesky critters away, create your own bug spray using the best insect-repelling oils. Here's how:

Ingredients

- 3 drops lemongrass oil
- 4 drops citronella oil
- 2 drops peppermint oil

Method

- Dilute with your favorite carrier oil.
- Add to a spray bottle and spray lightly on your skin if you're going outside.
- Avoid citrus oils such as orange and lemon as they can be phototoxic.

Blend #4: Sunburn Relief

Few things are as enjoyable as a day in the outdoors soaking up the sun. However, too much UV exposure can lead to sunburn. And for some, this can be quite painful. The good news is that you can make a soothing blend that will provide you with instant relief!

Ingredients

- 5 tbsp coconut oil

- 8 drops tea tree oil
- 8 drops of lavender oil
- 8 drops peppermint oil
- 1 cup aloe vera juice

Method

- Add all ingredients to a dark glass spray bottle.
- Shake well to combine.
- Spray on affected areas as often as your skin feels burning or itchy.
- It's a good idea to spray this mixture onto your skin after a bath or shower and before bed.
- You can also add some of this blend (or a tea tree and carrier oil mixture) to your bath water for added relief.

Blend #5: Winter Immunity Booster

Stocking up on vitamins is especially necessary in the cooler months as we head into winter. However, that is often not enough to keep cold and flu symptoms at bay. With that in mind, adding an immunity-boosting blend to your arsenal goes one step further in fighting viruses.

Ingredients

- 1 drop eucalyptus oil
- 1 drop lavender oil
- 1 drop rosemary oil
- 1 drop of sweet orange oil

- 1 drop of tea tree oil

Method

- Add all these oils to your diffuser.
- Let the diffuser run for about 30 minutes in the room you're in.
- Do this several times per day.

Blend #6: Peaceful Sleep Blend

A good night's rest is essential to our overall well-being. However, the stresses and pressures of daily life often take their toll and make sleep near impossible. If you're struggling with your sleeping patterns, it's a good idea to create a blend with a few oils that are known for their calming and soothing properties.

Ingredients

- 2 drops of chamomile oil
- 2 drops of lavender oil
- 2 drops of ylang-ylang oil

Method

- Mix oils and add to your diffuser.
- Let the diffuser run for about 30–60 minutes as you unwind and get ready for bed.
- If you meditate or do a yoga session before bed, this is the perfect time to run your diffuser.
- You can also add a carrier oil to the above mixture, use the whole solution in a spray bottle, and then lightly spray your pillows and

sheets about an hour before bed. I've found that coconut or olive oil is a great carrier oil option for this purpose.

Blend #7: Body Pain Relief

If you frequently suffer from body aches or muscle pains, it can be challenging to find the right medication, especially if you're experiencing these aches and pains in different places. Essential oils such as lavender, peppermint, and oregano have amazing anti-inflammatory properties that soothe inflammation and reduce swelling.

Ingredients

- 1 tbsp of coconut oil or your favorite carrier oil
- 2 drops of lavender oil
- 4 drops peppermint oil
- 3 drops oregano oil
- 3 drops of cedarwood oil

Method

- Mix all the ingredients and place the mixture in a dark bottle.
- Apply the blend to any painful or swollen areas.
- This blend is also great for adding to a foot spa or bucket of warm water if you have swollen feet.
- Keep in mind that coconut oil has excellent anti-inflammatory effects, making it a top choice as a carrier oil.

Blend #8: Essential Oil Chest Rub

Another way to combat the effects of winter is to rub a soothing vapor rub into a sore and congested chest, especially if the scent instantly opens your chest. Now, making your own chest rub involves a few extra steps, but it's still easier than you think.

Ingredients

- 2 tbsp coconut oil
- 2 tbsp unscented shea butter
- 6 drops peppermint oil
- 6 drops eucalyptus oil
- 2 drops rosemary oil

Method

- Bring a pot of ¼ cup of water to a slow boil over medium heat with a double boiler.
- Add the shea butter and coconut oil into the double boiler.
- Stir every few minutes to melt and mix the butter and oil.
- Once the mixture is completely melted, remove from the heat and let rest.
- As soon as the mixture has cooled down but not hardened, add the oils and mix well.
- Transfer to your dark jars and let cool.
- Rub on your chest two to three times per day.
- It's a good idea to rub some on your chest just before bed to aid with breathing while you're sleeping.

Blend #9: Diffuser Cough Blend

No one likes a nagging cough. And, since cough syrup isn't exactly on anyone's favorite medicine list, it may be a good idea to try a wonderful antibacterial blend that will soothe your airways and help you get rid of your cough.

Ingredients

- 3 drops wintergreen oil
- 2 drops rosemary oil
- 3 drops frankincense oil
- 4 drops eucalyptus oil

Method

- Add the oils to your diffuser.
- Let the diffuser run in the room for 30–60 minutes at a time.
- Be sure to diffuse about 30 minutes before bed to reduce coughing during the night.

Tips to Integrate Essential Oil Blends Into Your Wellness Routine

In my own experience, I've found that the most effective way to include essential oils into your daily life is by integrating them into your wellness routine. Not only will you get the many benefits of essential oils, but you'll also get to enjoy them while treating yourself to some much-needed self-care. On that note, we're next going to look at a few of the top ways you can incorporate your freshly made essential oil blends into your daily self-care routine.

1. **Add Your Essential Oil Blend to Your Face Cream**

Certain essential oils have excellent benefits for your skin. This makes adding your favorite blend to your face cream a great way to incorporate these oils into your self-care routine. Keep in mind that you have two options here—you can choose to add your top blend to the whole jar of cream or you can scoop out the amount you need every day and mix it with a different blend.

However you go about it, adding a blend to your face cream allows you to give your skin exactly what it needs every day. Personally, I prefer to do it this way to avoid adding different blends to my jar of cream. Here are a few oils that are perfect for adding to your face cream:

- carrot seed oil (boosts healthy-looking skin)
- frankincense oil (reduces the appearance of uneven skin tones)
- copaiba oil (cooling and refreshing and reduces the appearance of blemishes)
- lavender oil (calming properties are excellent for night cream)

2. **Create a Sugar Scrub**

Sugar scrubs are a wonderful, natural way to gently exfoliate your skin. Combining your favorite blend with coconut oil or shea butter will leave your skin beautifully soft. Another enormous plus point is that a sugar scrub is quick and easy to create, making it great for beginners. Here's a simple sugar scrub recipe you'll want to add to your self-care routine:

- **Ingredients**
    - ½ cup brown or white sugar
    - 1 tbsp coconut oil
    - 2 tbsp grape seed or jojoba carrier oil

- - 5–10 drops of lavender essential oil (you can substitute this with peppermint, rose, or even chamomile oils if you prefer)
  - dried lavender (optional)
- **Instructions**
  - Mix the sugar and oils.
  - Add dried lavender flowers and mix gently.
  - Transfer to a glass jar.
  - Use as needed.

Keep in mind that the fragrance of the carrier oil you choose may affect the scent of your scrub. Grape seed has the mildest scent which makes it a popular choice here.

3. Add a Refreshing Blend to a Hot Bath

A hot bubble bath after a long day is one of the best ways to unwind and relieve muscle aches and stress. Adding a few drops of your favorite blend to your bath water is also a quick and effective way to incorporate oils into your wellness and self-care routine. Here are a few essential oils that are known for their calming effects:

- lavender (calming effect)
- ylang-ylang (calming and moisturizing)
- peppermint (eases nervous tension and sore muscles, and opens chest congestion)

Remember to dilute your chosen essential oil with a carrier oil such as almond, coconut, or even jojoba.

4. **Use Essential Oils to Your Massage Routine**

Whether you're massaging tired, sore feet or getting a massage from someone else, you may want to include your favorite blend as part of your pampering session. Here, the only precaution is that you should tell the person giving you the massage what's in your blend to avoid an allergic reaction. Now, the most common oils to opt for in a massage routine include these:

- lavender (obviously)
- cedarwood (boasts many relaxing properties)
- peppermint (is invigorating and energizing)
- eucalyptus (boosts alertness)

5. **Add a Few Drops of Essential Oil to Your Diffuser**

Diffusing oils is an excellent way to enjoy the benefits of your blends, clear the air in your space, and avoid a potential allergic reaction. It's also an amazing way to absorb your oils if you're too busy for a massage or a long, hot soak. Here are a few of my favorite diffuser blends that you may want to try:

- **Energize blend:** I use this citrus blend to get me focused for the day.
    - 2 drops lemon oil
    - 2 drops orange oil
    - 2 drops grapefruit oil
    - Dilute with a carrier oil of your choice.
- **Stress blend:** Have a stressful, hectic day to deal with? Well, I use this stress blend in my office on such occasions:
    - 2 drops lavender oil

- 3 drops bergamot oil
- 2 drops frankincense oil
- Dilute with a carrier oil of your choice.

- **Calming blend:** Everyone can benefit from a calming blend wafting through the home or office—it's a great way to boost your mood and calm nerves.
  - 2 drops lavender oil
  - 2 drops peppermint oil
  - 2 drops lemon oil
  - Dilute with a carrier oil of your choice.

- **Bedtime blend:** If you struggle to fall asleep, maintain healthy sleeping patterns, or have insomnia in general, it's a good idea to add lavender to your diffuser. As a natural sleep aid, lavender will help you relax, which can then, obviously, help you fall asleep. Start diffusing about four to five drops of lavender 30 minutes before bedtime to boost relaxation.

6. Create a Sinus Steam Bath

Very few things can be as annoying and uncomfortable as a stuffy, congested nose. Whether your symptoms are related to seasonal allergies or a bout of the flu, you'll be delighted to learn that the right essential oil can provide relief!

Just as lavender is famous for its calming properties, eucalyptus is well-known for its benefits in respiratory health. This is why it's such a common ingredient in flu and allergy medicine. A quick way to ease a stuffy nose or congestion is by having a sinus steam bath a few times a day. On that note, here's how can create the perfect sinus bath:

- The best essential oils for sinus congestion are eucalyptus, peppermint, tea tree, clary sage, oregano, lavender, and even rosemary.

- Add three to seven drops of one of the above essential oils to boiling water in a heatproof bowl or large pot.

- Cover your head with a towel and take deep breaths in through your nose, inhaling the steam.

- Only do this for about two to five minutes at a time.

- Repeat a few times throughout the day and at night before bed.

7. **Add Essential Oil to Your Meditation or Yoga Sessions**

Another fun way to incorporate your newly created blends into your wellness routine involves adding them to your meditation or yoga sessions. Indeed, doing this creates a relaxing atmosphere and encourages mental alertness. Here are a few of the best ways to incorporate your oils into your next yoga or meditation session:

- Opt for a relaxing blend to use in your diffuser in the space where you practice yoga or meditate.

- Add a few drops of your diluted blend to a cotton ball or tissue and inhale deeply before you begin your session.

- Apply diluted oils to your temples, pulse points, or the soles of your feet. This is an excellent way to ground yourself, setting the perfect tone for an effective meditation session.

- Spritz a few drops of your favorite, diluted oil onto your yoga mat, helping you to relax.

8. **Use Essential Oil Blends Around the Home**

Not all mental stressors happen out in the world. Sometimes, allergies, a stuffy room, or stale air can aggravate your overall wellness. To counter this, use essential oils to cleanse the air in your home. And yes, there'll be more about this in the next chapter!

Now, one of the most appealing reasons for using essential oils is that there's no shortage of recipe blends to try out. Whether you want to make a simple two-oil mixture for mild headaches or create a much more complex mixture for a chest rub, there are so many different oils to consider using. When one type of mixture doesn't work, you can always substitute one of your oils for another! Just be sure to make notes of your different blends so that you remember exactly how you made the ones you've found the most useful.

With that said, it's time to head into Chapter 6, where we'll take a closer look at the many ways in which you can use essential oils around your home and office. From incorporating the oils into your cleaning products to keeping pests away, the next chapter is well worth a read!

Chapter 6:

Using Essential Oil Blends Around the Home and Office

Aromatherapy conveys the concept of healing with aromatic substances.
–Robert Tisserand

If you're anything like me, then you're always looking for ways to use less harsh chemicals around the house. For the most part, this is because the ingredients in some commercial cleaning chemicals, air fresheners, and insecticides can be quite harmful to your health. Furthermore, some of these chemicals can also be detrimental to the environment.

Of course, finding organic cleaning methods is nothing new. But if you're exploring the green cleaning concept for the first time, you'll be pleasantly surprised to learn that essential oils are a wonderful and effective alternative to a cupboard full of risky chemicals. With that said, where does one start? How do you know which oils are best for certain tasks? Well, this chapter is going to answer those questions, and more than that, it's going to share a bunch of wonderfully easy recipe blends that you can mix up in no time!

The Benefits of Using Essential Oils Around the Home

Honestly, there are so many benefits to using essential oils around your home. Whether you're using oils only to cleanse the air or relying on their antibacterial properties to replace commercial cleaners, there's no denying that your home environment will benefit. Here are a few of the top benefits you can look forward to:

- **Toxin-free:** The number one driving force behind the green cleaning concept is using fewer toxins. Since essential oils are either made from cold pressing or distilling plant components such as leaves, roots, flowers, or seeds, there's no adding of harsh or toxic chemicals. This is a huge benefit, as many of the chemicals used in commercial cleansers often contain ingredients that create or aggravate respiratory symptoms.

- **Multipurpose:** If you only use commercial cleansers around your home, chances are you have a whole cupboard or shelf full of bottles, each with a specific purpose. You may have cleaners for the kitchen, bathroom, and bedrooms, as well as stain removers, oven cleaners, carpet cleaners, window cleaners—the list goes on! Essential oils such as tea tree and eucalyptus have high antibacterial properties, which makes them excellent multipurpose options for use on a variety of surfaces.

- **Antiviral and antibacterial properties:** When you're cleaning spaces such as your kitchen and bathroom, you'll want solutions that neutralize bacteria, viruses, and other harmful pathogens. Oils such as peppermint, lemon, and tea tree oil easily remove dust mites, bacteria, and mold. Sweet orange oil, on the other hand, is excellent for degreasing surfaces, making it a wonderful option for cleaning cutting boards and countertops.

- **Aromatherapy benefits:** While some people may not mind their homes smelling like bleach and cleaning products, I personally prefer a home that has a more natural, soothing scent. Furthermore, strong-smelling commercial products often give off fumes that can irritate your eyes, cause headaches, or even aggravate asthma symptoms. Thankfully, combining your favorite essential oil with cleaning marvels such as vinegar and baking soda is an excellent way to enhance the aroma in your home. Indeed, the scent of essential oils will not only create a calming atmosphere but also promote relaxation and improve your overall mood!

Top Tips and Recipes to Use Essential Oils Around Every Part of Your Home

Understanding the benefits essential oils offer is only the first step. As with the medicinal uses discussed in the previous chapter, I must point out that to get optimal results from your blends, you need to use the right oils for each job. To help you with this, here's a list of tips containing the most effective blends that my own family uses around our home:

Tip #1: Use Essential Oils to Clean Counters and Surfaces

Keeping your kitchen counters and tables clean and grease-free is crucial to maintaining a healthy cooking and eating area—not to mention keeping bugs out. However, you may not always want to spray harmful cleaning aids on the same counters on which you prepare your family's meals. So, it's time for a natural solution.

Ingredients

- 5–10 drops of orange oil (you can use both the wild and sweet versions)
- 30ml carrier oil such as jojoba or almond oil
- Enough baking soda to create a paste (depends on the amount of cleaning you want to do)
- ¼ cup vinegar (this will depend on how much you want to make)

Method

- Mix the oils and create a paste with the vinegar and baking soda. (Here, you want to create an abrasive paste that will help the orange oil remove grease and stubborn residues)

- This mixture is ideal for use on ovens, countertops, stovetops, tables, and even sinks.

- Orange oil is well known for its degreasing properties, and combining it with vinegar and baking soda (which are also top natural cleaning and antibacterial agents!) makes for a magic cleaning solution.

Tip #2: Add Cotton Balls to Your Cupboards

Ever noticed how some cupboards can develop a stale smell, especially if you don't open them often? Without a doubt, essential oils are the secret to keeping your cupboards smelling fresh.

Ingredients

- a few drops of your favorite essential oil (options with a stronger fragrance such as eucalyptus or lavender are a good idea)
- cotton wool balls

Method

- Add a few drops of your chosen oil to the cotton wool balls.
- Place the cotton wool balls in the corners of your cupboard.
- Add a few drops to the balls as soon as they feel dry and the scent seems to be fading.
- Choose a scent you like, as this fragrance will transfer to the items in the cupboard.

Tip #3: Add to the Tumble-Dryer to Fragrance Your Clothes and Linens

If you're looking for a quick way to add fragrance to your clothes, linens, and even curtains, then the answer is to do it while the items are in the tumble dryer.

Ingredients

- 5–10 drops of lavender oil
- a carrier oil of your choice

Method

- Mix your essential oil with a carrier oil such as jojoba or grapefruit.
- Add a few drops of the mixture to a small cloth or terry towel and place it in your dryer with the items with which you want to infuse the scent.

Tip #4: Refresh Your Carpets

Carpets are wonderful—they can be aesthetically pleasing, comfy on the feet, and ideal for keeping your home warmer in the winter. However, keeping them clean and smelling fresh can prove quite challenging. Fortunately, one of your blends might just do the trick!

Ingredients

- 10 drops of peppermint oil (you can use any essential oil, but peppermint is a natural deodorizer, making it a great choice for clearing away carpet odors)
- 200 grams of baking soda

Method

- Mix the peppermint oil and baking soda and place them in an airtight container. Let the container sit for about two days before using it. This will ensure that the oil isn't clumpy.

- After two days, open the container, and stir well to ensure the oil and baking soda have mixed well.

- Sprinkle this homemade carpet powder on your carpets and let sit for a few hours.

- Vacuum the carpets.

- Enjoy your fresh-smelling carpets, and repeat as often as necessary.

Tip #5: Eliminate Pet Odors

If you have pets living in your home, then you're likely familiar with the annoying aspect of pet odors. And while you may currently be putting oil in the diffuser to neutralize the air, it might be time to give the floor a good sanitizer.

Ingredients

- 10 drops of lemongrass, geranium, or eucalyptus oil (all of these are excellent for eliminating pet odors)

- 30ml of carrier oil such as jojoba, coconut, or olive oil

- half a bucket of hot water

Method

- Add the drops of your chosen oil to the bucket of hot water.

- If the stain or odor is strong, consider creating a blend made up of two oils, one of which is eucalyptus, as it's also a strong sanitizer.

- Wash the area where the odors are strongest.

- If the area is carpeted, wash the carpet with this solution, and once dry, sprinkle with the powder created in Tip #4.

Tip #6: Create Your Own Air Freshener

Another commercial product that's a common staple in every household is an assortment of air fresheners. Have you given any thought to the ingredients in these aerosol cans or plastic spray bottles? Suffice to say, it may be time to clear the air with a more natural product.

Ingredients

- 10–20 drops of essential oils with a fragrance you enjoy such as lavender, peppermint, lemon, or eucalyptus

- 30–50ml carrier oil of your choice (grapefruit and coconut oil are good options to enhance the scent of your essential oil)

- Distilled water or witch hazel to fill the bottle

Method

- Mix your essential and carrier oils with distilled water or witch hazel.

- Add to your spray bottle and mix well before use.

- Spray the mist around your home the same way you would your store-bought air freshener.

- Using an oil such as lavender will also act as a mood booster.

Tip #7: Add a Blend to Your Vacuum Cleaner

A home with carpets requires extensive vacuuming. Ever thought of fragrancing your carpets or rugs while vacuuming?

Ingredients

- 2–5 drops of your favorite essential oil (use the same oil you're using for your air freshener to avoid conflicting aromas)
- a few small pieces of thin tissue paper

Method

- Bundle up the thin tissue paper and add the oil drops.
- Suck the tissue up with your vacuum.
- Since the tissue is now inside the vacuum, it will start dispersing a wonderfully invigorating aroma around your home.
- Citrus oils and lavender work well for this.

Tip #8: Neutralize Kitchen Odors

The average kitchen is filled with a range of different aromas. Finding a natural solution to rid your kitchen of cooking odors can be challenging. However, as with everything else, the secret lies in using the right oil.

Ingredients

- 5–10 drops of any spice oil such as clove, cinnamon, or cardamon
- a large pot

Method

- Place a pot of water on the stove until it simmers.
- Add the essential oil you've chosen.
- Be sure to use an oil from the spice category if you want to mask kitchen odors.

Tip #9: Eliminate Tobacco Odors

Tobacco odors can be quite annoying in a home where not everyone is a smoker. It can also be quite overwhelming for visitors. As such, making the right blend will help neutralize any tobacco odors.

Ingredients

- 5 drops of rosemary
- 5 drops of pine
- 5 drops of thyme
- 30ml carrier oil of your choice (I like grapefruit for this, personally, as it doesn't overwhelm the other oils in this blend)

Method

- Mix all the oils and add them to your diffuser.
- Run the diffuser in various rooms throughout the day.
- Remember to keep pets and children out of the areas where you're running the diffuser, especially if you're running it for extended periods.

Tip #10: Create a Window Cleaning Solution

Commercial window cleaning solutions are effective, but they can also leave you with a headache. When it comes to embracing the green cleaning concept, opting for a natural window cleaner is a great leap forward.

Ingredients

- 5–10 drops of orange oil
- 5–10 drops of eucalyptus oil

- 30–50ml carrier oil such as jojoba or coconut
- 1 cup of white vinegar (this will depend on the amount of solution you want to make)
- distilled water

Method

- Mix your oils with the vinegar and distilled water and add to your spray bottle.
- Spray the solution onto the windows and wipe off with a clean, microfiber cloth to prevent streaks.
- Keep in mind that using a citrus oil such as orange not only lifts any dirt or grease but also deters potential bugs who want to fly in.
- Note, too, that vinegar is an antibacterial agent, and as such, it's excellent for cleaning stubborn dirt.

Tip #11: Restore Wooden Furniture

If you're cleaning or trying to restore wooden furniture, you should never do it with a harsh chemical solution. These chemicals can strip the natural sheen of the wood and leave them looking dull.

Ingredients

- 5–10 drops of lemon oil
- 30ml olive oil
- distilled water

Method

- Mix the oils with the distilled water and add to your spray bottle.

- Add this mixture to your wooden furniture to clean and revive the shine.

- You can also add linseed oil to your mixture, as this is also an effective wood treatment.

Tip #12: Revive the Grout in Your Floor and Wall Tiles

There's no need to spend hours and bottles full of commercial cleaners trying to get the grout between your tiles clean. Give this a whirl instead!

Ingredients

- 5 drops of orange essential oil (this oil is great for cleaning away grease and stubborn dirt)

- enough baking soda to make a paste (this may depend on the size of the area you're cleaning)

- ¼ cup vinegar (again, this may be more or less depending on your area)

Method

- Add the orange oil (pine oil is also a good option) to the baking soda and vinegar, and create a paste.

- Apply the solution to the grout lines and let sit for a few minutes to draw out the dirt and grease.

- Scrub if necessary and wash the area with a damp cloth or mop.

- You can also add a few drops of oil to the water that you're using to rinse the area.

Tip #13: Freshen Your Mattress

Mattresses are another household item that can be difficult to keep clean and fresh. However, with an essential oil solution, it's easier than you think.

Ingredients

- 5–10 drops of lavender oil (this can be more if you're making a large mixture to freshen all the mattresses in your home in one cleaning session)
- enough baking soda to sprinkle on your mattress

Method

- Mix the essential and carrier oils.
- Sprinkle the baking soda over your mattress, as this will help to neutralize any odors.
- Spray the lavender oil mixture over your mattress and let it sit with the baking soda. Leave for anywhere between a few minutes to a few hours, depending on the state of the mattress.
- Vacuum the baking soda up. You can spray another layer of lavender oil over the mattress before adding the bedding. This will promote a restful night's sleep.

Tip #14: Neutralize Bathroom Odors

When it comes to dealing with odors, the bathroom more than likely tops your cleaning list. And I'm sure I don't have to tell you that spraying commercial chemicals often doesn't help. So, it may be time to opt for a natural and healthier solution.

Ingredients

- 3–5 drops of lemon oil

- 3–5 drops of pine oil
- 3–5 drops of lavender oil
- 30ml carrier oil
- cotton wool balls

Method

- Mix the essential oils with the carrier oil.
- Add a few drops of this mixture to the cotton wool balls.
- Place the cotton wool balls discretely around your bathroom for optimum effect.
- Ensure that you place them in covert spaces where children and pets can't reach them.
- You can also use this solution—or the one in Tip #6—to create a bathroom air freshener if you prefer a spray to cotton wool balls.

Tip #15: Freshen Your Shoes

Shoes are often high on the list of odor offenders in the typical home. In addition to regularly cleaning them and ventilating them outdoors, you can also create a natural solution to keep them smelling fresh!

Ingredients

- 3–5 drops of an odor-masking essential oil such as cinnamon, cedarwood, tea tree, or lemon
- 30ml carrier oil such as jojoba, almond, or olive oil
- ¼ cup vinegar (this would depend on the amount of solution you need)

Method

- Mix the oils and vinegar in your spray bottle.
- Use a damp cloth to wipe out the shoes.
- Lightly spray the inside of the shoes.
- Don't spray too much, as this can pool in the shoes and risk damaging the soles.
- Once you wipe the mixture out of the shoes, air dry them in the sun if possible.

Tip #16: Remove Mold and Mildew

Moisture-prone areas such as the kitchen, bathroom, and laundry room are also at risk of developing mold and mildew. And not only is this unsightly, but these bacterial spores can also lead to severe respiratory illnesses. Fortunately, there's a natural solution to this common problem.

Ingredients

- 5–10 drops of tea tree oil
- 5–10 drops of eucalyptus oil
- 5–10 drops of lavender or citrus oil
- 30ml carrier oil such as olive, jojoba, or almond
- enough vinegar to fill your spray bottle (if you have a very big bottle and don't want to fill it, only add as much vinegar as you think you'll need)

Method

- Combine all the oils with the vinegar and mix well.
- Spray the area where you have seen mold or mildew spores.

- Let sit for a few minutes.

- Scrub the mold from the area and wash it down with hot, soapy water. You can even add a few drops of tea tree oil to your cleaning solution to sanitize the area.

- If you're dealing with a tough mold spot or a particularly large area, be sure to wear gloves and a mask to avoid inhaling the spores as you scrub.

- Regularly clean that area with a tea tree solution, as this should keep mold spores from returning while you address the underlying cause.

Using Essential Oils to Repel Bugs Around Your Home

No matter where you live, chances are that you're occasionally dealing with some seasonal pests or bugs around your home. And not only are they annoying, but they can actually spread disease and contaminate open food sources. While numerous so-called "home-safe pesticides" can be used to rid your space of these pesky bugs, it's important to be mindful of the dangers that are often associated with these poisons. They are *poisons,* after all!

Now, many people are wary of using essential oils as a form of pest control, and this mainly comes down to the natural element. Indeed, the general belief is that only a *chemical* can eliminate pests. But guess what? That's simply untrue. So how, then, can you use essential oils to get rid of bugs? Let's find out!

How Do Essential Oils Deter Pests?

First of all, keep in mind that essential oils are made from *plant components.* So, in their natural form, these components repel predatory insects in order to keep the plant safe. When these plant parts are crushed into oils, these same components are still active in the solution. As it turns out, oils with strong scents are excellent for blocking a bug's odorant receptors, which would normally attract them to various aspects of your home.

To me, this sounds like a top reason to include a few insect-repellent options in your list of must-make blends! And as such, I've compiled a few suggestions below that I've had the most success with.

Two Top Mosquito Blends to Try

If you live in a hot, humid area, then you're no stranger to the swirling irritants that are mosquitoes—especially in the summer months. And if you're looking for a chemical-free way of deterring these pests, the good news is that there are a few essential oil blends that should do the trick!

Mosquito Blend #1: Citronella Oil

Citronella oil is one of the most effective essential oils used to repel mosquitoes. In fact, you may recognize the name from candles and other natural products geared at keeping mosquitoes at bay. Indeed, citronella works because it affects the insect's olfactory receptors, which simply means they can't smell you. And if they can't smell your natural carbon-based scent, chances are they won't find you as appetizing as before.

Ingredients

- 10–20 drops of citronella oil (use 10 drops if you're making a solution for a small bottle and 20 drops if you're using a much bigger spray bottle)
- 30ml of your favorite carrier oil
- 100ml distilled water

Method

- Mix the citronella, carrier oil, and distilled water together, and add the mixture to a spray bottle. Adding the distilled water makes more of a solution than simply using the oils only, especially if you want to make a larger quantity. Some users even prefer to use vodka in place of distilled water, which provides you with the added antibacterial benefit of the alcohol.

- Spray the solution around your patio, garden, or any area with a lot of mosquito activity.

- The best time to spray is at dawn or dusk, however, if you have a water feature near your patio, you may find that they're active all day.

Mosquito Blend # 2: Lemon Eucalyptus

If you can't find a bottle of citronella oil, you can also opt for a combination of lemon and eucalyptus oils, as this makes for another potent mosquito repellent. Now, I should point out that this is especially a great alternative for people who have a citronella allergy. You can use olive oil as a carrier, but you can also use vodka, distilled water, or even witch hazel to fill your spray bottle.

Ingredients

- 10–20 drops of lemon oil
- 10–20 drops of eucalyptus oil
- 30ml of your favorite carrier oil
- 100ml distilled water, vodka, or even witch hazel

Method

- Mix the oils, carrier oil, and distilled water and add to your spray bottle.

- Spray the solution in the air around your patio or wherever you've seen mosquito activity.

- You can also mix the lemon and eucalyptus into a fragrance-free cream such as shea butter to create a topical lotion that can be applied to the skin. This is handy if you're sitting outside in an area where the mosquitoes are buzzing around.

- Experts have found that eucalyptus oil can be effective for up to three hours, making it a great blend to try (Frances et al., 2014).

Blends to Keep General Household Pests Away

Of course, mosquitoes aren't the only pests that invade our homes or office spaces. Other pests such as ants, roaches, spiders, and mice can also infest our spaces, spreading disease, and causing damage to furnishings or wooden structures. Not to mention, they even invade our pantries and grocery cupboards!

Thankfully, you don't have to create a specific blend for each insect. Instead, you can create a simple essential oil spray suitable for use on *all* of these bugs you've seen scurrying around. Here are a few well-worth making:

Pest Deterrent # 1: Peppermint Oil

While *you* may enjoy the sweet, candy-like smell of peppermint oil, most common household pests don't find the smell quite so appealing. In fact, the menthol component is a well-known deterrent because of its biocidal properties that easily destroy mites, mosquitos, and other pests.

Ingredients

- 10–20 drops of peppermint oil

- 30ml of carrier oil (peppermint oil works well with jojoba or almond oil)

- 100ml distilled water

- vinegar or alcohol to top up your spray bottle

Method

- Mix your oils with the distilled water and the alcohol.
- Shake well before use.
- Spray the solution on the surfaces where you've seen the bugs.
- It's a good idea to spray some of this solution on door frames as well as the corners of your home.

Pest Deterrent #2: Lavender

Lavender isn't just good for calming your nerves and helping you get some much-needed rest in the evenings. That's right—it's also a superb deterrent for a host of insects! The component linalool found in lavender is especially useful in deterring flies.

Ingredients

- 10–20 drops of lavender oil
- 30ml of carrier oil (lavender oil works well with jojoba or almond oil)
- 100ml distilled water
- vinegar, witch hazel, or alcohol (such as vodka) to top up your spray bottle

Methods

- Mix the oils with the water, vinegar, or alcohol.
- Add to your spray bottle and spray in areas where you've spotted the pests. Be sure, again, to include the entry points to your home.

- An added advantage of using lavender oil is that it also gives your home a soothing aroma.

Pest Deterrent #3: Tea Tree Oil

If your pest problem is a little *closer* to a family member's skin—if you follow me—then you may want to try a tea tree blend. Indeed, when it comes to neutralizing head lice, tea tree oil is an excellent choice—the same goes for its ability to prevent lice eggs from hatching.

Additionally, a tea tree solution can be used to get rid of ticks and fleas on your pet's bedding! Just remember, though, as discussed in Chapter 2, that pets may have a very bad reaction to essential oils. That means you'll have to spray the bedding *away* from where your pets usually sleep and wash or sterilize their bedding to remove any traces of the tea tree oil once the bugs have died.

Ingredients

- 10–20 drops of tea tree oil
- 30ml of carrier oil (tea tree oil works well with almond, olive, or avocado oil)
- 100ml distilled water
- vinegar, witch hazel, or alcohol (such as vodka) to top up your spray bottle

Method

- Mix the oils with water, vinegar, witch hazel, or alcohol.
- Add to your spray bottle. For bedbugs, spray this solution on mattresses, sofas, and carpets.
- If you're treating head lice, you can add the tea tree and carrier oil directly to the shampoo that you'll be using.

Using Essential Oils Around the Office or Workspace

Once you start using essential oils, I guarantee that you'll quickly learn how wonderful they are for your overall health and wellness. And this may leave you wondering just how you can incorporate them into every aspect of your life, including, of course, your work life!

Whether you work in a space away from home or have a home office, making use of a few of your essential oil blends is a great way to deal with everything from stress to boosting mental clarity.

Top Reasons to Use Essential Oils in Your Workspace (And the Blends to Help You Do It)

In addition to simply loving the effect essential oils have on your space, there are a bunch of credible reasons as to why adding a blend or two to your work environment is a smart move. I've listed the most significant below:

It Creates a Clean Workspace

There's no denying that workspaces have their fair share of germs and bacteria floating around. And this is especially true if you work in an open-plan office environment where everyone has access to your desk, phone, keyboard—even your stapler! Thankfully, using a tea tree, eucalyptus, or even sweet orange blend is an excellent way to keep the germs at bay. Here's how:

Ingredients

- 10 drops of sweet orange
- 10 drops lavender

- 15 drops of your favorite carrier oil
- ¼ cup vinegar

Method

- Mix the oils and vinegar and add to a spray bottle.
- Spray counters and table tops and wipe down with a damp cloth.
- Don't spray the solution onto electronic components or display screens. Instead, spray the blend onto a clean, damp cloth and wipe down your computer screen, keyboard, desk phone, and other items.
- Be sure to store your blend away from direct sunlight, preferably in a dark cupboard, and clearly label it to avoid accidental ingestion.

It Purifies the Air

Of course, germs and odors don't just settle on our workstations. They can also hang around in the air, putting everyone at risk of allergies or illness. And this is especially the case during flu season. As such, the best way to reduce the number of pathogens, germs, and bacteria floating around in your office is to add a diffuser to the space. Indeed, using a diffuser is often the best way to disperse the oil blends all over the office, just as you would at home. If you get the go-ahead from your colleagues, try starting with a simple lavender or tea tree blend. The top oils that are known for their air-purifying qualities include the following:

- tea tree
- cinnamon
- lavender
- clove
- rosemary

- oregano
- thyme

It Reduces Stress

No matter how relaxing your workplace may be, there will be days when everything just seems to be going crazy all at once. For some work environments, a stressful environment simply goes with the territory. Nonetheless, your space is sure to benefit from a daily stress-reducing blend. Once again, add an oil or blend created with soothing oils to the office diffuser.

Without any doubt, a calmer workspace is not only good for business but beneficial to everyone's health as well. The most common oils to use to create a stress-reducing blend include the following:

- lavender
- sandalwood
- chamomile
- ylang-ylang
- frankincense
- bergamot

Use the same ratio as the blend in the first point of this section. You can use one oil and a carrier, or you can create your own blend using a few of the oils listed above. Just remember not to use oils that overpower each other to avoid creating headaches.

It Boosts Productivity

Workplace tension and negative energy are huge contributors to low work morale. So, one way to keep these low feelings from creeping up on everyone is to opt for a few blends made of oils that boost morale, promote optimism, and enhance feelings of well-being. Adding the right oils to your work diffuser will get everyone in a better mood. Here are a few to try:

- rosemary
- lemon
- frankincense
- wild orange
- lavender
- peppermint
- jasmine

It Works in First Aid Treatments

Typically, every office space should have a regulated first aid kit. However, if your workspace is your home office, it's a good idea to have a blend on hand that can be used for minor first-aid treatments. In this instance, it's a good idea to opt for oils with the most effective antimicrobial and antiseptic properties. Create a few first-aid blends using the following oils:

- **Lavender:** Can be used for headaches, insect stings, and minor burns.
- **Tea tree:** Great for sunburn, as well as cleaning cuts and scrapes.
- **Helichrysum:** Excellent for assisting with swelling, bruising, and sprains when applied as part of a cold compress.
- **Lemon:** Wonderful for the treatment of minor cold and flu symptoms.

As you can see, essential oils are great for more than just medicinal purposes. Incorporating your favorite blends into both your home and office spaces is another simple way to ensure that you get optimal results from essential oils. As well, opting to use your blends rather than the harsh chemicals found in commercial cleansers is a great choice in reducing your and your family's exposure to harmful chemicals.

Now, despite the simplicity of using essential oils, it's important to point out that mistakes can and do happen. That's why, as we move into Chapter 7, I'm going to be sharing with you a few of the most common beginner mistakes, as well as the best ways to avoid them. So, keep reading, and let's get acquainted with the do's and don't of blending your favorite oils!

Chapter 7:

Essential Oil Mistakes to Avoid and Troubleshooting Blending Mishaps

> *There are many different oils that have a beneficial effect on your mind.*
> —Amy Leigh Mercree

As you begin exploring and applying essential oils to every aspect of your life, it's important to be aware of the few things that often can and *do* go wrong. While trial and error is an important part of learning what works best for you, knowing what errors you can avoid in the first place will go a long way toward avoiding allergies and exposing yourself or your family to potential toxins.

So, this chapter is going to take a look at a few of the most common mistakes beginners encounter on their journey to creating a successful blend. Additionally, I'll be sharing a few troubleshooting tips to help you deal with beginner mistakes.

Essential Oil Mistakes to Avoid

At their core, essential oils are remarkably potent. And when they're combined with other oils to make blends, their potency can increase quite significantly. With this in mind, it's important to understand that some oils, when blended, can become toxic, and as a result, do more harm than good. So, if you want to get the best—and safest—results from your essential oils, blends, and their subsequent applications, be sure to avoid the following beginner mistakes!

Mistake #1: Not Taking the Time to Learn About Essential and Carrier Oils

Courtesy of the internet, many people are under the impression that doing comprehensive research on essential oils is *unnecessary*. After all, you can just Google as you go, right? Wrong. It's crucial to take the time and make the effort to learn as much as you can about essential oils before you start purchasing ingredients for your first blend.

Make a point of learning about what each oil is best used for, how they should be diluted, and more importantly, what the safety precautions and side effects are. Doing this will ensure that you create, store, and apply your oils and blends in the safest way possible. Furthermore, it will also ensure that you don't waste money buying items you may not need.

Mistake #2: Buying Poor-Quality Oils

As you'll recall, I highlighted this point back in Chapter 1—and yes, it's important enough to stress again here. Please, avoid buying poor or low-quality oils. Believing that all essential oils are the same no matter what brand you buy is an unsafe assumption to make.

While the oil itself may be the same, some brands opt to use fillers and additives to make up the quantity required to fill the bottle. Simply put, they're watered down. Not only is the expected quality compromised but the fillers and additives may cause or aggravate allergies and other negative effects.

The golden rule is to always opt for 100% organic or pure essential oil. The best places to find quality oils are aromatherapy stores, health food stores, or certified online sites. And remember, genuine essential oils will always have an informative label and detailed information on the manufacturer's website.

Mistake #3: Not Using a Carrier Oil

Just because you've never had a negative reaction to an essential oil doesn't mean you can ditch the carrier oils when it comes to topical applications. While this may work out for *some* oils, combining them in blends increases the risk of burning and rashes if used in their pure form.

When you're setting up your first starter kit, be sure to include a few different carrier oils to experiment with. For most blends, you can use the carrier oil of your choice. Keep in mind, though, that some may affect the end fragrance, which means you need to opt for a milder option. The most common carrier oils to consider include the following:

- grapeseed oil
- rosehip oil
- sweet almond oil
- coconut oil
- jojoba oil
- olive oil
- apricot oil
- hemp seed oil

Mistake #4: Running Your Diffuser All Day and Night

Once you start using your oils in a diffuser, you will find that your home smells amazing and everyone's mood seems improved. These positive results may lead you to want to leave your diffuser on 24/7. After all, since essential oils are natural products, doesn't this mean that we can use them as much as we want?

The reality is that constant exposure to diffused essential oils can create headaches or aggravate existing respiratory illnesses such as asthma. As such, a safer alternative is to leave your diffuser on for 30—60-minute intervals and then switch it off. As well, ensure that the room is well-ventilated so that you don't create an instance of overexposure to the oils. Lastly, if you often forget to turn your diffuser off, opt for a model with a timer that you can preset.

Mistake #5: Leaving the Lids Off the Essential Oils

Leaving the lids off essential oil bottles as you create your blends is a common beginner mistake. This practice may be fine with baking ingredients, but when it comes to your oils, it's outright unsafe. As I mentioned in Chapter 2, essential oils are made up of different components that can turn to vapor if they're exposed to oxygen for too long. This will cause your oils to start evaporating and at the same time deteriorate their quality. So, try to work slowly and replace the lid of each bottle as soon as you have extracted the drops you need.

Mistake #6: Using Your Pointer Finger to Dab On Your Blend

This is a mistake that I learned the hard (and painful) way! If you're using your index finger to rub your essential oil onto your temples or anywhere else, it becomes very easy to forget about the oil on that finger afterward—and before you know it, you're accidentally rubbing or scratching an itchy eye. Needless to say, this can cause a burning sensation.

To avoid this, use a cotton swab or cotton wool ball to apply your blend topically. So, rather than dab your temples with your pointer finger, the idea here is to use *something else* to do the dabbing. Alternatively, teach yourself to use a finger that you would *never* use to rub or scratch your eye. Either way, get into the habit of washing your hands before and after each blend creation and application.

Mistake #7: Ingesting Essential or Carrier Oils

As part of your initial research, you may read a wide variety of articles on essential oils and their uses. That's great and all, but some of these articles may suggest ingesting certain oils in the case of certain ailments. Now, I would caution against this—especially for beginners. This is because ingesting oils that haven't been blended correctly can lead to serious side effects or cause serious damage to your body. Make no mistake, applying your oils or blends topically is a much safer and more holistic way to enjoy the benefits of essential oils.

Mistake #8: Forgetting That Some Oils Can Stain

While it's true that the telltale sign of a quality essential oil is that it's less likely to stain, the reality is that, ultimately, they are just *oils*. And, well, oils tend to stain. This is particularly true when it comes to the following oils:

- chamomile
- jasmine
- tangerine
- myrrh
- patchouli

As a rule of thumb, I treat all oils as if they stain. This forces me to be careful about how I apply them, and I also ensure that I massage them into my skin properly to avoid exposure to clothes.

Mistake #9: Applying Oils That Are Photosensitive and Then Going Outside

This mistake usually happens when newbies are excited to create a bug spray or when they include it in their lotions to avoid sunburn. Keep in mind that some oils, especially those in the citrus family, are *phototoxic*. This means they will react to the sun, and as a result, increase your UV sensitivity. Ultimately, this will lead to redness, burning, itching, and overall irritation. So, when creating a topical blend or one that you're going to mix into your creams, avoid the following oils:

- sweet orange
- lime
- lemon
- tangerine
- grapefruit
- bergamot
- cumin
- mandarin

Mistake #10: Using Oils and Blends Around Your Pets

Many essential oils are helpful for conditions that our pets also experience. Despite this, you should never be tempted to apply or even spray essential oils near your dogs or cats. While some people may argue that there are oils you can use safely on a dog's skin, this would depend on the oil, its concentration, the pet, and its existing medical history. If your pet has a condition that you think will benefit from a drop or two of essential oils, it's imperative to discuss this with your dog's vet first.

Troubleshooting Essential Oil Blending or Application Issues

Sadly, undesirable reactions are not uncommon when you start creating your essential oil blends. As with everything else, learning to make safe and effective essential oil blends takes considerable practice. However, if you've made a mistake with your blend or the way you're applying your oils, there is usually a way to rectify the situation. Below, I've listed a few of these trial-and-error moments that may require some troubleshooting.

Troubleshooting Tip #1: My Blend Is Burning My Skin

The problem: Applying your blend or diluted essential oil has caused a burning sensation on your skin.

The cause: There are a few reasons why oils could be burning your skin. Here are a few of the top causes:

- You have applied the essential oil without diluting it with a carrier oil.

- Your skin is sensitive or you may be allergic to that particular oil.

- The oil blend you have created may be made up of one or a few "hot" oils. Spicy oils such as clove, cinnamon, oregano, thyme, cassia, and lemongrass are known to cause a burning sensation on sensitive skin.

The solution: To overcome itchy skin from your essential oil blend, consider the following:

- To create immediate relief, apply some olive or coconut oil to the area.

- Always dilute your essential oils with a carrier oil. The top options are coconut, olive, jojoba, and almond oil.

- Follow the dilution guidelines in Chapter 3 to get your blends diluted correctly. If you have sensitive skin or you're using a spicy oil, you may need to add a little more carrier oil.

- If you're adding a blend to a cream or lotion, don't add the blend to the whole container of cream (in case an allergic reaction occurs). Rather, scoop the cream into a different container and then add a bit of the blend to test.

- Do a skin patch test for every new blend you create. While you may not be allergic to essential oils overall, your skin may be sensitive to the combination of the oils you have added to the blend. Put some of the blends on a small area to test your skin's tolerance.

- Be sure to stick to recommended essential oil quantities. For sensitive skin or stronger oils, consider using a few drops less.

Troubleshooting Tip #2: My Blend Is Giving Me a Rash

The problem: A rash has developed on your skin immediately after or a few hours after applying a blend.

The cause: When a rash occurs on your skin, it can be attributed to one of the following aspects:

- The oils you have used are having an adverse reaction to the accumulated synthetic chemicals trapped in the fatty layers of your skin.

- You have used too many essential oils and not enough carrier oil in your blend.

The solution: A rash can be as annoying as having itchy, burning skin. Here's what you can try:

- Add more carrier oil to your blend. You can start with a ½ teaspoon at a time.

- Reduce the number of oils you're adding to your blends. Typically, start with two oils at a time.

- Use fewer drops of oil as you mix the blend, especially the stronger oils such as eucalyptus.

- Reduce the time between applications. For instance, instead of applying the oil every two hours, apply it every four hours instead.

- Drink more water to eliminate any accumulated toxins from your skin. It's a good idea to shower or bathe before applying the blend to avoid rubbing dust or sweat into your skin, which can also create a rash.

Troubleshooting Tip #3: I Accidentally Got Oil in My Eye

The problem: You've accidentally got oil in one or both eyes and they are burning and watering.

The cause: Getting essential oils in one or both eyes usually happens when you have been working with or applying your blends and then accidentally rubbed your eyes. Alternatively, you may have applied some oil to your temple for treatment of a headache and some has run into your eye. (Yes, it happens!)

The solution: Fortunately, this is one of the easiest mistakes to treat and avoid. Here's how:

- For immediate relief, don't rub your eyes. Instead, saturate a tissue with a carrier oil such as olive, coconut, or jojoba oil and place it on the affected eye. This will help neutralize the essential oil.

- While rinsing your eye with water might be your go-to method, keep in mind that many essential oils don't mix with water, which means the water won't wash the oil out.

- Don't apply essential oils directly to your eyes or the immediate area around the eyes.

- Never apply your headache blend while you're lying down, as a few drops can easily roll down from your temples into your eyes. Also, be sure to thoroughly massage the oil into your temples.

- Always wash your hands after working with your oils and blends. Having some oil on your fingers can easily end up in your eyes if you suddenly reach up to scratch an itch.

- Get into the habit of applying your essential oils with cotton wool or a Q-tip to avoid getting any on your fingers. Alternatively, you can avoid using your index finger to apply your oils. As the finger that most people use to rub their eyes, it's often the culprit in accidental eye applications.

Troubleshooting Tip #4: My Essential/Carrier Oil Has Stained My Clothes

The problem: Your essential oil blend or carrier oil has left a stain on your clothing, curtains, carpet, or furniture.

The cause: Dark-coloured essential oils are more likely to stain fabrics and materials. Typically, this has to do with the additional pigments found in darker oils which are difficult to eliminate. Alternatively, the blend has been left to sit on a particular fabric or furniture item for too long.

The solution: Oil stains can be very difficult, if not impossible to remove. Keep these tips in mind:

- An immediate solution is to soak up as much oil blend as possible using a white paper towel.

- Familiarize yourself with the types of oil that are most likely to stain. Typically, these are the darker oils such as cinnamon, tangerine, and myrrh.

- Keep in mind that lighter oils may also stain if they are left on the fabric for too long.

- If you're going to use oils on clothes, curtains, or other fabrics, do a patch test on a small piece of material first.

- Where possible, avoid using oils on your clothes or reduce the quantity of oil used in the blend and applied to the material.

- To remove the stain, try the following:
    - Dampen the material with lukewarm water.
    - Create a paste with baking soda and warm water and apply to the stain.
    - Scrub with a sponge or toothbrush and let sit for 30–60 minutes.
    - Rinse the paste away. Repeat if necessary.
    - Keep in mind that this may not work on all types of material.

Troubleshooting Tip #5: My Blends Don't Seem to Be Working

The problem: It can be very disheartening when your essential oil blends aren't working. And this is especially true when someone else seems to be having resounding success with the exact same recipe blend.

The cause: There are many reasons why your essential oil blend may not be giving you the desired results. Here are the most common reasons to look out for:

- Your blend is overconcentrated. Essential oils work if the right amount is added to the blend for the intended purpose. Too much can actually leave you feeling *worse*. This can also happen if you're leaving your diffuser on for too long. So, yes, in the case of essential oils, you can have too much of a good thing.

- You're using the wrong oil. Not all oils are created equally, and the oil you've chosen may not have the right properties to deal with the ailment or issue at hand.

- Application is irregular. For oil blends to work, they need to be applied consistently.

- You expect too much of your oil blend. Essential oils should be used as part of a holistic practice, not as a singular cure for an ailment.

The solution: To avoid being disappointed with your blend, consider the following tips:

- Don't create an overconcentrated oil blend. Start small and test your body's tolerance to the various blends. Be sure to record any instances that aggravate your symptoms so that you can tweak your next blend.

- Sick to the 30–60 minute rule for your diffuser time. If you feel worse after a diffuser session, consider leaving the unit on for a shorter period. Be sure to have a window open in the area to ensure proper ventilation.

- Use the handy index table you're about to see in Chapter 8 to find the right oil for your ailment. Since most ailments have several oils that can be used, it's easy to find an alternative if a specific oil is not working or is causing an allergy. So, be sure to choose an oil for its particular healing properties rather than its lovely fragrance.

- Apply the blend as recommended. Using the blend once every few days may not be as effective as applying it daily or twice daily. Of course, keep in mind that the blends may require several applications to take effect. It's also important to note—once more—that not all oils work equally well for everyone. While lavender might make you sleepy, it may do absolutely nothing for someone else. So, test small quantities of the oils related to your ailment and see which one works best for you.

- Speak to a professional aromatherapist, as the level of your ailment may require a specialized synergy blend.

And there you have it! Those are, for my money, the most common mistakes to avoid, paired with some troubleshooting tips that will benefit your essential oil journey for years to come. Ultimately, remember that it all starts with creating the right blend for the ailment or household issue you want to resolve.

Whether you want to get rid of a pesky headache or clean your kitchen counter, there's an oil for you. And by using this list of mistakes to avoid and troubleshooting tips, your essential oil journey will be considerably easier! Now, onward to Chapter 8, where, as I've mentioned already, you'll be met with an index table that I hope you find as helpful as I do!

Chapter 8:

Handy Index Table

I expect that essential oils may someday prove a vital weapon in the fight against strains of antibiotic-resistant bacteria. –Dr. Andrew Weil

As you've already learned by now, essential oils can be used for quite a wide variety of ailments. However, what happens when you can't find stock of a specific oil or you have an adverse reaction to it? Well, thankfully, you don't have to give up on your essential oil journey if you're faced with either of those issues. As you'll see, this chapter is dedicated to offering you the following handy index table. In it, I've carefully compiled a few oils that can be used for some of the most common ailments.

This way, if you can't find a specific oil, have an allergic reaction to a certain one, or simply don't like a particular fragrance, you can opt for another one on the list! I've actually printed this table out and stuck it on the wall of my workspace where I create my blends. It makes the process so much easier, so feel free to do the same!

Ailment	Essential Oils	Precautions
Acne	<ul><li>Bergamot</li><li>Camphor</li><li>German chamomile</li><li>Cistus</li><li>Juniper</li></ul>	<ul><li>Avoid using camphor during pregnancy</li></ul>

Anxiety	- Basil - Roman chamomile - Clary sage - Jasmine - Lavender	- Avoid using basil during pregnancy
Arthritis	- Sweet birch - German chamomile - Peppermint - Eucalyptus	- Avoid using sweet birch during pregnancy
Bronchitis	- Allspice - Cedarwood - Clove - Cypress - Eucalyptus	- Don't use on children younger than two years
Irritable bowel syndrome	- Caraway - Coriander seed - Dill - Fennel - Marjoram	- Don't use on children younger than two years - Oils are for massaging on the affected area only

Chills	• Allspice • Black pepper • Grapefruit	• Grapefruit is phototoxic
Chest congestion	• Sandalwood • Cedarwood • Thyme • Eucalyptus	• Don't use on children younger than two years
Coughing	• Allspice • Thyme • Sandalwood • White tea tree • Cedarwood	• Don't use on children younger than two years
Circulatory conditions	• Geranium • Laurel leaf • Rose • Thyme • Ylang-ylang	• Don't use on children younger than two years
Colds	• Star anise • White tea tree • Eucalyptus	• Don't use on children younger than two years

	• Clementine • Frankincense	
Constipation	• Cardamom • Celery seed • Dill • Mandarin • Orange • Peppermint	• Don't use on children younger than two years • Oils are for massage purposes
Cystitis	• Basil • Bergamot • Cedarwood • Eucalyptus • Sandalwood	• Don't use on children younger than two years
Dental and teething	• Chamomile • Laurel leaf	• Don't use on children younger than two years • Oils are for massage purposes only
Digestive tract conditions	• Aniseed • Basil • Celery seed	• Avoid during pregnancy and lactation

Fatigue	• Black pepper • Thyme • Allspice • Spearmint • Peppermint • Jasmine	• Don't use on children younger than two years
Flatulence	• Allspice • Spearmint • Rosemary • Ginger • Clove	• Don't use on children younger than two years • Oils are for massage purposes only
Fungal infections	• Cinnamon • Citronella • Tea tree • Lemon balm	• Don't use on children younger than two years
Fever	• Eucalyptus • Citronella • Lemongrass • Bergamot	• Don't use on children younger than two years

Gout	<ul><li>Angelica root</li><li>Juniper</li><li>Pine</li><li>Rosemary</li><li>Spruce black</li></ul>	<ul><li>Don't use on children younger than two years</li></ul>
Headache	<ul><li>mjAnise</li><li>Basil</li><li>Chamomile</li><li>Sage</li><li>Eucalyptus</li></ul>	<ul><li>Don't use on children younger than two years</li></ul>
Head lice	<ul><li>Myrtle</li><li>Eucalyptus</li><li>White tea tree</li><li>Balsam of Peru</li></ul>	<ul><li>Don't use on children younger than two years</li></ul>
Insomnia	<ul><li>Lavender</li><li>Bergamot</li><li>Chamomile</li><li>Sage</li><li>Nutmeg</li><li>Sandalwood</li></ul>	<ul><li>Don't use on children younger than two years</li></ul>

Indigestion	• Turmeric • Allspice • Peppermint • Cardamom • Chamomile • Lemon balm	• Don't use on children younger than two years • Never ingest these oils (refer back to Chapter 2 for safety precautions)
Insect bites	• Rosewood • Lemongrass • Lemon • Lavender • Eucalyptus	• Don't use on children younger than two years
Intestinal spasm	• Tarragon • Turmeric • Cinnamon Leaf • Fennel • Lemongrass	• Don't use on children younger than two years
Immune system tonic	• Cinnamon bark • Thyme • Douglas fir	• Don't use on children younger than two years • Oils are for massage purposes only

Joint stiffness	- Allspice - Tea tree oil	- Don't use on children younger than two years
Menstrual cramps	- Basil - Clary sage - Cypress - Dill - Eucalyptus - Geranium	- Don't use on children younger than two years
Muscular aches	- Ginger - Hyssop - Laurel leaf - Lavender - Lemongrass	- Don't use on children younger than two years
Mouth ulcers	- Lemon - Myrrh - Orange	- Don't use on children younger than two years
Nausea	- Allspice - Basil - Chamomile - Clove	- Don't use on children younger than two years - Oils are for massage purposes only

Nervous exhaustion	- Ginger - Tangerine - Sandalwood - Sage - Rosemary - Pine - Patchouli	- Don't use on children younger than two years
Promote hair growth	- Grapefruit - Rosemary	- Grapefruit is phototoxic
Parasitic infections	- Basil - Camphor - Cinnamon - Clove - Eucalyptus	- Don't use on children younger than two years
Rashes	- Camphor - Lavender - Chamomile - Citronella - Niaouli	- Don't use on children younger than two years

Relaxing	• Lavender • Sandalwood • Bergamot	• Don't use on children younger than two years
Respiratory infection	• Cedarwood • Eucalyptus • Oregano	• Avoid oregano during pregnancy or lactation
Rheumatism	• Allspice • Angelica root • Basil • Birch • Cedarwood • Chamomile	• Don't use on children younger than two years
Stress	• Allspice • Basil • Bergamot • Cedarwood • Chamomile • Grapefruit	• Grapefruit is phototoxic
Sore muscles	• Bergamot • Gingergrass	• Don't use on children younger than two years

Skeletal inflammation	• Sweet birch	• Avoid during pregnancy or lactation
Sinus	• Ginger • Eucalyptus • Cedarwood • Camphor • Peppermint	• Don't use on children younger than two years
Sunburn	• Chamomile • Lavender • Tea tree	• Don't use on children younger than two years
Tension	• Valerian • Sandalwood • Nutmeg • Rosemary • Rose geranium • Lavender	• Don't use on children younger than two years
Urinary tract infection	• Cedarwood • Frankincense • Juniper • Copaiba	• Don't use on children younger than two years

Varicose veins	- Celery seed - Geranium - Lemon - Peppermint - Rosemary	- Don't use on children younger than two years
Viral infections	- Oregano - Lemon balm - Clove - Cinnamon - Thyme	- Avoid oregano during pregnancy and lactation

Conclusion

Every essential oil has a healing purpose, so I think it's a great gift because it's something that elevates your mood and your health. –Yolanda Hadid

Ultimately, there are many reasons why you may want to embark on the essential oil blending journey. Whether it's to uplift your mood, embrace the green cleaning concept, or take a more holistic approach to your general well-being, trust me—you're making the right choice. Essential oil blending can have a positive effect on your life in so many ways.

When I started my own journey, I found that it was often very time-consuming to gather all the information needed to create safe and healthy blends. More than once I found myself thinking that it would be so much easier if all the information I needed was compiled in an easy-to-understand, user-friendly guide. And, since I couldn't find one that provided all the information I needed, it hit me—the next logical step was to create one!

And with that, I set out to create a guide that not only showcased the wonders of essential oils but also shared a few helpful recipes, tips, and guidelines. Here at the end, I hope I have succeeded in offering you exactly that. To highlight the top pointers from this guide, though, let's recap what exactly this guide has shared:

Understanding the Basics

When you first decide to explore the exciting world of essential oil blending, it's imperative to start researching everything you need to know about the oils you want to use. This involves knowing the difference between essential and carrier oils as well as knowing whether an oil is a top, middle, or base, along with how it affects your ultimate blend.

For your convenience, I added a list of common names accompanied by their scientific names. Having this list to refer back to will ensure that you know precisely what oil you're dealing with when you're creating your starter kit. And, of course, opting for quality oil is the key to successful and safe blends.

Heed the Precautions

Despite being among the top holistic approaches, essential oils should only ever be used once you understand the precautions surrounding their use. This includes using the right oil for a specific purpose. So, be sure to heed the precautions discussed in Chapter 2 to avoid suffering an allergic reaction.

Getting Started

Getting started is all about gathering the right equipment. With so many essential oils on the market, my list of the top 12 is a good place to start. That said, knowing how you're going to apply your blends is crucial before you really get blending. Be sure to stick to the guidelines about blending as well as the tips on safe dilution processes. Keep in mind, too, that if a current dilution is burning your skin, this usually means you should increase your carrier oil. I included a conversion table that will help you create your blend no matter what system your recipe is in.

Choose the Right Technique

Choosing the right blending technique will make getting started much easier. Being aware of the various techniques also gives you different options to try. A big tip from me here? Don't be afraid to experiment with a few unconventional oils, especially when you're creating blends to help treat common ailments. And once you have found a favorite supplier, be sure to check out their synergy blends.

Therapeutic Benefits

The primary reason many people start creating essential oil blends is the amazing therapeutic benefits one can expect. If blended and used correctly, you will be able to treat everything from a mild headache to a bout of sunburn. Just be sure to label your blends by mentioning what's in the bottle and what it was created for. For instance, "Tea Tree/Lavender - Sunburn Solution."

So Many Home Uses

Essential oils and the blends you create are not only wonderful for treating a variety of ailments but they also have extensive uses around the home. The right blend will not only clean and freshen your carpets but also keep your kitchen counters germ-free! Furthermore, essential oils are a simple and effective way to get on board with the green clean concept. Indeed, with the right oil blends, you can reduce the amount of harsh chemicals being used in your home without sacrificing your hygiene standards.

Beginners Mistakes

Every new journey is filled with a trial-and-error process. In fact, blending mistakes are not uncommon, even for experienced essential oil users. On that note, knowing what mistakes can happen will make it easier to avoid them. Additionally, having a few troubleshooting tips in hand will help you fix any blending or application errors.

Handy Index Table

Back when my journey began, and I was going about my initial research, another aspect I found lacking was a comprehensive list of the types of oils one can use for various ailments. I found this especially frustrating in instances where there would only be one oil listed per ailment, and that particular oil was out of stock from my local supplier. Needless to say, having a list of alternative oils makes creating blends so much easier!

And Lastly...

I have thoroughly enjoyed sharing what I have learned about the wonders of essential oil with you. While it may seem overwhelming in the early days when you're trying to gather equipment, oils, and recipes, the good news is that—as with everything else—it gets easier with practice. Start small, be sure to source quality products, and keep detailed notes of your blends, favorite brands, and recipes. Also, never be afraid to tweak your recipes to suit your needs, and be patient with yourself as you embark on this fun and insightful journey.

And with all that said, let me close off by wishing you all the best on your journey to embracing the wonders of essential oils. Happy blending!

If you have found this guide helpful and informative, I urge you to leave a positive review and share how the tips you've learned here have helped you on your essential oil blending journey. In doing so, you will make it considerably easier for other people on the same journey to find this guide!

About the Author

With a global background spanning Singapore, New York, London, and Sydney, Clara deBeyer is an environmental science professional and corporate consultant. Over the past five years, she has navigated both her interest in the changing environment we live in and the complexities of corporate consulting. Beyond her consultancy role, Clara also showcases an entrepreneurial spirit through successfully running her own photography business. Family is central to Clara, who balances a professional life with raising three children and their beloved four-legged companion. Outside work, she finds solace in nature, enjoying ocean swims, beach walks, and a passion for travel. While Clara is adventurous with food, she humbly admits that culinary skills might not be her forte. Her global travels have cultivated an appreciation for diverse cuisines and passion for trying new things. Motivated by curiosity and an open mind, Clara explores ways to enhance her quality of life. This journey led her to scent psychology, discovering the impact of essential oils on mood during a challenging period of grief. Embracing change and innovation, Clara is a perpetual learner dedicated to personal growth and improving both her life and the lives of those around her.

References

Alek Ashunk. (2020, July 13). *Top, middle & base note essential oils with blending chart.* Lavenderandoil.com. https://lavenderandoil.com/essential-oil-notes/

American College of Healing Sciences, E. T. (2016, September 16). *5 delightful and work-enhancing essential oils for the office | achs.edu.* Info.achs.edu. https://info.achs.edu/blog/best-essential-oils-for-the-office

AromaTools®. (2019, August 4). *Essential oil troubleshooting.* AromaTools®. https://aromatools.com/blogs/aromatools-essential-ideas/essential-oil-troubleshooting

Bedosky, L. (2023, March). *Essential oil do's and don'ts: Aromatherapy tips for beginners.* EverydayHealth.com. https://www.everydayhealth.com/wellness/essential-oil-dos-and-donts-aromatherapy-tips-for-beginners/

Bio Source Naturals, A. T. (2022, June 5). *Essential oils & ten biggest mistakes you can make.* Bio Source Naturals. https://biosourcenaturals.com/essential-oils-ten-biggest-mistakes-you-can-make/

Bohinen, S. V. (2023, September 5). *Top 20 essential oil recipes.* Volant Europe. https://volantaroma.com/blogs/recipes/top-20-essential-oil-recipes

Brown, A. (2023, September 25). *Essential oils vs. carrier oils: Understanding the difference and benefits.* Www.linkedin.com. https://www.linkedin.com/pulse/essential-oils-vs-carrier-understanding-difference-benefits-brown

Camille. (2024, February 6). *The power of essential oils for cleaning | Natural Solutions. The Mag* 'Wecasa. https://www.wecasa.co.uk/mag/essential-oils-for-cleaning/

Chaffin, J. (2020, January 30). *How to substitute essential oils.* Plant Therapy; Plant Therapy. https://www.planttherapy.com/blogs/blog/how-to-substitute-essential-oils#:~:text=For%20example%2C%20most%20citrus%20oils

Checklistmaids. (2023, April 4). *5 benefits of cleaning with essential oils | Brooklyn Cleaning Service.* Checklist Maids Queens NYC. https://checklistmaids.com/5-benefits-use-essential-oils-cleaning-home/

Christine. (2024, February 24). *How to create your own essential oil blends.* Blog.mountainroseherbs.com. https://blog.mountainroseherbs.com/how-to-blend-essential-oils

Cronkleton, E. (2019, August 9). *How to use essential oils with a diffuser, on the skin, in bath, more.* Healthline. https://www.healthline.com/health/how-to-use-essential-oils

Dec. 01, K. E., & 2023. (2023, December 1). *What to know about natural cleaning products and which ones to use.* Family Handyman. https://www.familyhandyman.com/list/natural-home-cleaning-products/

Dr. Josh Axe. (2019, April 5). *Essential oils: 11 main benefits and 101 uses - Dr. Axe.* Dr. Axe. https://draxe.com/essential-oils/essential-oil-uses-benefits/

Essence of Thyme Editorial Team, E. (2023, February 15). *The top aromatherapy tools you must have.* Www.essenceofthyme.com. https://www.essenceofthyme.com/blog/top-aromatherapy-tools--must-have

Essentials, A. (2021, February 1). *Why aren't my essential oils working?* Abbey Essentials. https://abbeyessentials.co.uk/blogs/news/why-aren-t-my-essential-oils-working

Farr, N. (2020, March 24). *Buying essential oils is like shopping for diamonds — Here's how to Spot a Fake.* Greatist. https://greatist.com/health/best-essential-oils-how-to-buy-essential-oils#how-to-identify-fake-oils

Farrar, A. J., & Farrar, F. C. (2020). Clinical aromatherapy. *Nursing Clinics of North America*, *55*(4), 489–504. https://doi.org/10.1016/j.cnur.2020.06.015

Ferguson, J. (2021, January 5). *Back to work: The best essential oils for a productive office! | Inspire Me Naturally.* Undefined. https://www.inspiremenaturally.com.au/blogs/news/best-essential-oils-for-office

Fields, A. (2017, July 31). *Essential oils uses for common ailments | Life Beyond Organic.* Lifebeyondorganic. https://lifebeyondorganic.com/essential-oils-uses-common-ailments/

Fisk, C. (2020, September 15). *How to blend essential oils | Base Formula.* Www.baseformula.com. https://www.baseformula.com/blog/how-to-blend-essential-oils

Frances, S. P., Rigby, L. M., & Chow, W. K. (2014). Comparative laboratory and field evaluation of repellent formulations containing Deet and lemon eucalyptus oil against mosquitoes in Queensland, Australia. *Journal of the American Mosquito Control Association*, *30*(1), 65–67. https://doi.org/10.2987/13-6366.1

Freshkin. (2019, October 7). *Essential oils blending guide.* Freshskin Beauty. https://www.freshskin.co.uk/blog/essential-oils-blending-guide/

Galper, A. (2022, January 18). *Carrier oils vs essential oils - what's the difference!?* Cliganic. https://www.cliganic.com/blogs/the-essentials/carrier-oils-vs-essential-oils#

Gomez, L. (2022a, June 27). *Top 10 best essential oils.* Nikura. https://nikura.com/blogs/living-well/top-10-best-essential-oils

Gomez, L. (2022b, September 30). *Essential oils blending guide.* Nikura. https://nikura.com/blogs/discover/essential-oils-blending-guide

Hart, Dr. R. (2020, March 25). *14+ Amazing essential oils to treat sunburn.* Gyalabs.com. https://gyalabs.com/blogs/essential-oils/essential-oils-for-sunburn

Healingscents. (2018). *Healingscents.* Healingscents. https://healingscents.net/blogs/learn/18685859-history-of-essential-oils

Health, A. (2023, August 4). *AbundantHealth4u.com.* Abundant Health. https://abundanthealth4u.com/

Hoffman, P. (2022, November 3). *Can essential oils expire? Understanding essential oil oxidation.* Young Living Blog - US EN. https://www.youngliving.com/blog/do-essential-oils-expire-oxidation/

Hoftun, D. (2023, August 7). *Aromatherapy at work.* Volant Europe. https://volantaroma.com/blogs/recipes/aromatherapy-at-work

Hot Oily Mama, E. T. (2018, February 6). *7 Common mistakes using essential oils - Hot Oily Mumma.* Hotoilymumma.com. https://hotoilymumma.com.au/essential-oils/7-common-mistakes-using-essential-oils/

Kilgore, C. (2019). *Wellness Center | THE WELL New York.* The-Well.com. https://www.the-well.com/

Lane, J. (2018, November 8). *Top 150 list of essential oils with free cheat sheet.* Loving Essential Oils; Loving Essential Oils. https://www.lovingessentialoils.com/blogs/essential-oil-tips/list-of-essential-oils-pdf

Lane, J. (2023a, January 13). *Essential oil diffuser blends for sleep - 10 DIY recipes for bedtime — Loving Essential Oils.* Www.lovingessentialoils.com. https://www.lovingessentialoils.com/blogs/diffuser-recipes/sleep-essential-oil-diffuser-blends

Lane, J. (2023b, November 28). *7 common essential oil mistakes you might be making — Loving essential oils.* Www.lovingessentialoils.com. https://www.lovingessentialoils.com/blogs/essential-oil-tips/essential-oil-mistakes

Living, Y. (2019a, March 22). *Storing essential oils: The dos and...* Young Living Blog; Young Living Blog. https://www.youngliving.com/blog/essential-oil-storage-the-basics/

Living, Y. (2019b, August 26). *New to essential oils? 15 oils for beginners.* Young Living Blog - US EN. https://www.youngliving.com/blog/new-to-essential-oils/

Living, Y. (2020, February 18). *Essential oils you've never used before | Young Living Blog.* Young Living Blog - US EN. https://www.youngliving.com/blog/8-essential-oils-youve-never-heard-of-until-now/

Lozanova, S. (2022, March 25). *10 relief remedies using essential oils.* Earth911. https://earth911.com/living-well-being/essential-oils-10-remedies/

Lyth, by G. (2022, August 26). *10 easy ways to use essential oils around your home.* Quinessence Aromatherapy. https://www.quinessence.com/blog/10-easy-ways-use-essential-oils-around-home

MacNeill, J. (2021, December 21). *10 ways to use essential oils around your home.* Escents. https://escentsaromatherapy.com/blogs/news/10-ways-to-use-essential-oils-around-your-home

Martinez, F. (2021, June 4). *12 ways to use essential oils to scent a room.* MOXĒ. https://bemoxe.com/blogs/news/12-ways-to-use-essential-oils-to-scent-a-room

MHS, E. J. (2021, April 23). *Essential oil recipes for sunburn.* Elevays. https://elevays.com/essential-oil-recipes-for-sunburn/

Monsuri. (2023, September 8). *The ultimate guide to essential oil recipes for every occasion.* Monsuri. https://www.monsuri.com/blogs/health-and-wellness/the-ultimate-guide-to-essential-oil-recipes-for-every-occasion

Nathalie. (2019, March 19). *12 frequent mistakes for beginners using Essential Oils.* Pacific Scents. https://pacificscents.com.au/mistakes-for-beginners-using-essential-oils/

New Directions , A. T. N. D. (2023, November 9). *Magic of synergy blends - what are synergy blends & how do they work.* Www.newdirectionsaromatics.com. https://www.newdirectionsaromatics.com/blog/products/the-magic-of-synergy-blends.html

New Directions Aromatics, A. T. (2022, June 8). *The theory & practice of essential oil blending.* Www.newdirectionsaromatics.com. https://www.newdirectionsaromatics.com/blog/articles/the-theory-practice-of-essential-oil-blending.html

New Directions Aromatics, N. (2024, February 2). *Blending and diluting essential oils – Tips for safety and comfort*. Www.newdirectionsaromatics.com. https://www.newdirectionsaromatics.com/blog/articles/blending-and-diluting-essential-oils.html

Nourished Essentials, E. T. (2021, March 1). *9 essential oil recipes, and how to make them*. Nourished Essentials. https://nourishedessentials.com/blogs/healthwellness/9-essential-oils-recipes

Ogletree, A. (2021a, June 15). *6 essential oils that can help repel bugs and pests*. Angi. https://www.angi.com/articles/essential-oils-pest-control.htm

Ogletree, A. (2021b, June 15). *6 essential oils that can help repel bugs and pests*. Angi. https://www.angi.com/articles/essential-oils-pest-control.htm

Paul Frysh. (2017). *Slideshow: Dos and don'ts of essential oils*. WebMD. https://www.webmd.com/skin-problems-and-treatments/ss/slideshow-essential-oils

Perry, N. (2014, June 23). *Homemade sugar scrub with brown sugar & coconut oil*. Perry's Plate. https://www.perrysplate.com/2014/06/homemade-body-scrub-brown-sugar.html

Phillips, J. (2019, October 3). *Essential oil conversions and dilutions*. Jenni Raincloud. https://jenniraincloud.com/essential-oil-conversions/

Pike, D., & 2022. (2024, February 21). *12 safe, smart ways to use essential oils around your home*. Family Handyman. https://www.familyhandyman.com/list/safe-smart-ways-to-use-essential-oils-around-your-home/

Plant Guru Admin. (2020, August 29). *DIY essential oil recipes to relieve body aches*. Plant Guru. https://www.theplantguru.com/page/diy-essential-oil-recipes-to-relieve-body-aches/

PlantLife, E. T. (2019, October 11). *Essential oil mistakes to avoid*. Plantlife. https://plantlife.net/blogs/aromatherapy/essential-oil-mistakes-to-avoid

President, D. P., ACHS Founding. (2018, March 9). *Blending 101: The art of pairing essential oils drop by drop | achs.edu*. Info.achs.edu. https://info.achs.edu/blog/blending-101-the-art-of-pairing

Pugle, M. (2018, August 24). *Are essential oils safe? 13 things to know before use*. Healthline; Healthline Media. https://www.healthline.com/health/are-essential-oils-safe

Salmo, M. (2023, October 22). *10 reasons you should use essential oils*. The Little Details Home + Office + Digital Organizing Studio. https://thelittledetails.com/our2cents/10-reasons-you-should-use-essential-oils

The Sandalwood Shop, E. T. (2023, May 23). *8 easy ways to use essential oils around your home*. The Sandalwood Shop. https://www.thesandalwoodshop.com.au/blog/lifestyle-tips/8-easy-ways-to-use-essential-oils-around-your-home/

The Scent Apothecary , A. (2023, April 3). *6 ways to use aromatherapy oils in your self-care routine*. The Scent Apothecary. https://www.thescentapothecary.com/post/6-ways-to-use-aromatherapy-oils-in-your-self-care-routine

Scott, R. P. W. (2005, May 1). *Essential oil - an overview | ScienceDirect Topics*. Www.sciencedirect.com. https://www.sciencedirect.com/topics/earth-and-planetary-sciences/essential-oil#:~:text=Essential%20oils%20are%20highly%20complex

Sonoma Lavender, A. T. (2023, September 18). *5 powerful essential oils for natural relief from headaches and migraines (And how to use them)*. Sonoma Lavender. https://www.sonomalavender.com/blogs/news/essential-oils-for-headaches#:~:text=A%20blend%20of%203%20drops

Starkey, L. (2023, January 4). *7 potent essential oils and how to use them for better self-care*. Nurture My Body. https://nurturemybody.com/blogs/our-blog/7-potent-essential-oils-and-how-to-use-them-for-better-self-care

Tessendorf, K. (2023, September 1). *Scent customization made simple: The ultimate essential oil blending guide*. Volant Europe. https://volantaroma.com/blogs/guides/essential-oil-blending-guide

Van Pelt, K. (2022, July 19). *Freshen up your home with these 9 tips for using essential oils*. MyDomaine. https://www.mydomaine.com/how-to-use-essential-oils-to-scent-a-room-5184206

Weiner, Z. (2018, July 5). *The 10 best essential oils that everyone should have in their collection*. Well+Good. https://www.wellandgood.com/10-best-essential-oils/

Wellness Center Admin, W. (2023, July 14). *Wellness Center of Plymouth*. Wellness Center of Plymouth. https://wellnesscenterofplymouth.com/the-ultimate-guide-to-understanding-essential-oils-a-comprehensive-overview/

West, H. (2019, September 30). *What are essential oils and do they work?* Healthline. https://www.healthline.com/nutrition/what-are-essential-oils

Wilson, D. R. (2020, August 20). *Do essential oils expire? Average shelf life and how to extend*. Healthline. https://www.healthline.com/health/do-essential-oils-expire#why-they-expire

YBTT, K. (2018, February 21). *Essential oils at work: 7 brilliant uses of EOs in the office.* YBTT. https://www.yourbodythetemple.com/essential-oils-at-work/

Yee, M. (2019, May 9). *Essential oil allergic reaction: symptoms, treatments, and prevention.* Healthline. https://www.healthline.com/health/essential-oil-allergic-reaction

Yolanda. (2020, October 29). *How essential oils can enhance your daily self care routine.* Put the Kettle On. https://putthekettleon.ca/how-essential-oils-can-enhance-your-daily-self-care-routine/

Made in the USA
Las Vegas, NV
20 November 2024